Pelvic Pain Clinic

Shauna Farabaugh

and Caffyn Jesse

erospirit

Caution: The content of this book is not intended in any way as a substitute for professional medical advice, diagnosis, or treatment. Always seek the advice of your physician or other qualified health provider with any questions you may have regarding a medical condition. Somatic sex educators are not psychotherapists or medical practitioners.

All illustrations for this book were created by S. Murali Shanmugam with Caffyn Jesse, © Caffyn Jesse, except for the image of the pelvic bowl in Figure 5 and the fascia in Figure 21 which are from the public domain. The original colour illustrations are available in the Kindle version of this book.

Contents

Table of Figures 5

Acknowledgments 7

Introduction 9

Befriending the Body **12**
   Cultivating Somatic Awareness Practice 14

Working in our Personal Learning Zone **20**

Pelvic Anatomy **21**
   Muscles of the Pelvic Floor..22
   The Boney Bowl of the Pelvis 27
   Homologous Genital Structures...30
   Genital Nerves...32
   Penis Anatomy 34
   Vulva Anatomy..41
   Describing Pain and Pleasure: Layers 48

Causes of Pelvic Pain..**49**
   Pelvic Scars and Fascial Adhesions **49**
   Pelvic Pain and Trauma..**55**
   Embodied Sex Negativity and Pelvic Pain **59**

Treatments **61**
   Touch-based Treatment **61**
      Precautions and Possibilities with Touch....................................61
      Working with the Fascia in the Pelvis..62
      The Pelvis and the Jaw..66
   Topical Treatments..**69**
      Bioavailable hormones 69
      Cannabis-infused coconut oil..70
      Castor Oil Packs..71
      How to Make and Use a Castor Oil Pack 72
   Exercises **75**

Fascial Stretch..75
Pelvic Bowl Dancing 76
"Kiss the Earth" Breath..78
Pelvic Tilts..78
Squats...79
Hump and Hollow..81
Elevator 82

Beyond Pain to Pleasure..84
Staying Connected to Sexual Pleasure ....
with Persistent Pelvic Pain 89
Redefining Sex..89
Explore pleasure with relaxation or lower levels of arousal..............90
Explore the sensual...90
Kink and Power Play..91
Pelvic Pain and Partnership..91
Mindful Masturbation 92
Make Room for Resistance 93

Bibliography and Resources....................................94
About the Authors...97

Table of Figures

Figure 1: Table of Somatic Sensations 16

Figure 2: Breath engages the whole body, including the pelvis.............23

Figure 3: Pelvic Mobility...24

Figure 4: The pelvic diaphragm from above 27

Figure 5: The boney bowl of the pelvis 28

Figure 6: Homologous Genitals...31

Figure 7: Pelvic Nerves Diagrammed 32

Figure 8: Pelvic Nerves Illustrated...33

Figure 9: Penis Anatomy, external parts..34

Figure 10: Penis anatomy, saggital view 36

Figure 11: External penis showing possible changes with arousal and
    engorgement 37

Figure 12: Cross-section of the penis, showing erectile tissue 38

Figure 13: Circumcision Styles 39

Figure 14: Pelvic floor muscles...40

Figure 15: Vulva anatomy, external parts...41

Figure 16: Vulva anatomy, saggital view..43

Figure 17: The erectile tissue of the vulva, unengorged and engorged.44

Figure 18: Possible changes to the external vulva with arousal and
    engorgement. 45

Figure 19: Muscles of the pelvic floor.................................46

Figure 20: Anal sphincters 47

Figure 21: Image of fascia 50

Figure 22: Figure showing (a) healthy muscle, (b) response to injury, and (c) fascial organization in chronic pain conditions.........................51

Figure 23: Pelvic adhesions..54

Figure 24: Consider the opening of the vagina or anus like the face of a clock...65

Figure 25: In the saggital plane the pelvis moves forward and backwards 76

Figure 26: In the frontal plane the pelvis moves up and down 77

Figure 27: In the horizontal plane, the pelvis rotates in and out...........77

Figure 28:Pelvic tilts...79

Figure 29: Wide-legged squats stretch the pelvic floor 80

Figure 30: Hump and hollow 81

Figure 31: Schematic frontal cross section showing levels of muscles in the pelvic diaphragm 83

Acknowledgments

We would like to acknowledge some of our teachers.
Ellen Heed brought scar tissue remediation to sexological bodywork in 2010 at the invitation of Joseph Kramer. Ellen's extensive teachings on anatomy and treatment are foundational for both Caffyn and Shauna.
Kristin Lang and Katie Spataro are somatic sex educators who specialize in the treatment of pelvic pain. Their teachings have had a huge impact on Caffyn and all their students.
The teachings of John Barnes on the principles of myofascial release and its gentle nature are important to our practices.
Our most important teachers have been our courageous clients, whose struggles and triumphs in dealing with the many components of pelvic pain inspire us every day.

This book was kindly reviewed in manuscript by Katie Spataro, and we are especially grateful for her important input.

Introduction

In our work as somatic sex educators, we see many people whose lives and relationships have been profoundly impacted by persistent pelvic pain. People suffer from pelvic pain that is considered to be a chronic medical condition or pain that goes unreported and undiagnosed. There are many prohibitions and cultural silences about sex, urination and defecation. There is so much shame surrounding genitals and genital touch. There is a lack of information and disregard by the medical community about tending to the pelvis postpartum. These factors affect the willingness and ability people have to speak about their pain as well as the accessibility of effective treatment.

There are hundreds of medical conditions that can trigger persistent pelvic pain. Some of diagnoses you may hear or receive are: hormonal conditions, infection, lichen sclerosis, cliterodynia, vulvodynia, vaginal atrophy, herpes, allergic and autoimmune responses, vestibulodynia, repetitive strain, fibromyalgia, endometriosis, orthopedic problems, coccydynia, pelvic inflammatory disease, painful bladder syndrome, interstitial cystitis, prostatitis, peyronie's disease, dyspareunia, vaginitis, cervicitis, prolapse, dysmenorrhea, vaginismus and various cancers. Surgeries, accidents, sexual violence, gender dysphoria, childbirth and uncomfortable sex can trigger persistent pelvic pain. While some medical diagnoses lead to immediate and effective treatment, other diagnoses (including dyspareunia - pain with sexual intercourse, vulvodynia - chronic vulvar pain, and nonbacterial prostatitis - pain or discomfort with urination, sexual arousal or ejaculation) have no specific effective treatment available through a doctor's office. These conditions affect huge numbers of people. Nearly three out of four women have painful sex at some time during their lives, according to the American College of Obstetricians and Gynaecologists. Chronic nonbacterial prostatitis affects up to 50% of men.[1] When gender-variant and transgender people suffer from pelvic pain, the failure of the medical community as a whole (thus far) to educate itself on gender variance regularly compounds the challenges people face in seeking diagnosis and receiving effective treatment.

Original medical conditions frequently become complicated with anxiety, depression and social isolation, as pelvic pain affects sexual pleasure and intimate relationships, and is soon felt in all areas of our lives.

Complicating the diagnosis and treatment of pelvic pain is the difficulty people have in describing specific symptoms to medical professionals. People often do not know their own anatomy and physiology. In the absence of information, experience and attention, the nervous system is actually impaired, and people really cannot feel the tissues of the pelvis with discernment. Specific pain can become generalized and overwhelming. We include information on anatomy and physiology that we hope will empower people when seeking medical diagnosis and treatment of pelvic pain. Mapping specific areas of pain and pleasure and giving them names can also be empowering when exploring self-touch for healing and pleasure, and when in dialogue with partners. When people do not feel empowered to talk with medical professionals and partners, every medical exam and sexual encounter can bring about more pain and additional layers of injury.

Trauma frequently plays a role in the experience of pelvic pain. Sexual violence, surgery and other injuries can create scar tissue that has long-lasting and cumulative effects. Physical scars are but one dimension of trauma treatment. Trauma can also have a systemic effect that worsens the experience of pain and leaves us feeling less resourced to deal with it. It is important to work with trauma-informed health care providers, to play with trauma-informed sexual

---

[1] Wise and Anderson, p. 39

[2] adapted from Peter Levine

partners, and to educate ourselves on how trauma affects our own nervous systems.

Touch is known to be effective in the treatment of pain, yet touch that can relieve pain and induce pleasure is rarely used in the treatment of pelvic pain. And there are real dangers - as well as opportunities - in practices that address pelvic pain with touch. Possibilities for self touch, touch from a partner or friend, and treatments from professional touch practitioners are discussed, with precautions and guidelines for those who wish to explore.

Various topical treatments can be used to actually support tissue health, rather than simply numbing pain. Exercises and visualizations can help to ease pelvic immobility and encourage a shift from pain to pleasure.

Caffyn has been affected by pelvic pain for more than three decades, and learning to address their own pelvic pain was a major factor in guiding them to the study and practice of somatic sex education. Shauna has practiced somatic sex education with a focus on addressing pelvic pain for many years, and she teaches pelvic pain treatment to students of somatic sex education.

This book is intended as a resource to inform, support and companion people who are dealing with persistent pelvic pain. In our personal experience and through our professional practice with many clients, we know it is possible to reorient towards feeling pelvic wellness and experiencing pelvic pleasure, even as we work to address pain.

Befriending the Body

The somatic sex educator's approach to pelvic pain is different from that of other health care practitioners in that:

- we work *with* and *through* the body to address concerns

- we strive not only for the resolution of pain but also for access to pleasure

- we acknowledge and engage pleasure as a *resource* for healing pelvic pain

The word somatic comes from the Greek word *somatikos*, meaning "concerning the body" or *soma*, meaning "the living body in its wholeness". Our use of the word somatic conceptualizes the body not as a static object, but as a living, dynamic intelligence that guides us if we pay attention. In the words of Alexander Lowen, the founder of Bioenergetics, "You are your body". Most of us in this modern moment have lost access to the body's communication and don't feel connected to or identified with our bodies.

Through somatic sex education we invite you to a deeper and more integrated relationship with your body. We are not asking you to eschew or denigrate your big, beautiful brain, but rather to empower the brain part of you to think with and through the body part of you. Thoughts, moods, body functions and body sensations are all dynamically interrelated. If you've felt alone in trying to "figure out" your pelvic pain, notice how it feels to consider that you have an "inner team" on your side. While your brain has access to loads of information, ideas and strategies for healing, your body has additional information and strategies that you perhaps haven't yet conceptualized. Just imagine what you can accomplish when you start to listen to and learn from each other!

It's an understatement to say that it can be challenging to trust the body when it's been a source of pain, perhaps for years. You may feel let down or betrayed by your body. You may feel like your body is a burden. You may genuinely and passionately dislike your body. You may have, in fact, been choosing to disconnect from your body in an attempt to feel the pain less. But the body is not an adversary to be overcome, a problem to be solved, or an entity to be tamed. When we choose to notice, feel, and connect to our bodies—to become more embodied—we will likely feel our pain more clearly. But we will also increase our access to pleasure, and our access to knowing what we need to thrive.

The techniques in this chapter invite us to create a different relationship with sensation. Sensation is the language of the body. The practice of noticing the sensations in our bodies is called somatic awareness. For some, learning to cultivate somatic awareness will feel easy. For others it will be challenging. Some people learn to speak a new language easily, and others struggle. Honour your personal pace and process. Remember that this is a practice, not a test, and give yourself permission to learn slowly.

Somatic awareness helps us feel our pain with more precision, and find a language to communicate about it with doctors and partners. We can learn to distinguish between types of pain (burning, stabbing, aching, fuzzy etc.) and levels of pain (0 being no pain -10 being unendurable pain) as well as the specific anatomical locations of pain. It supports our personal sense of well-being when we notice and give articulation to "pain" as intricate and varied sensation, rather than one big overwhelming feeling. Pain is usually a complex series of specific sensations of different intensities, and these vary over time. With attention, we may also find pleasurable pelvic sensations, perhaps less intense, and in unexpected locations. Thanks to neuroplasticity, when we attend to what is pleasurable, our capacity for pleasure expands (see more on this in the following chapters).

By cultivating somatic awareness, we can learn to separate pain from the emotions and stories it generates for us. In giving the cascade of sensation within our bodies our attention and respect, we can simply feel the sensations of pain without immediately spiralling into stories about pain as inhibiting/diminishing/bad and wrong. Just noticing how sensations can be differentiated from thoughts, beliefs and emotions gives us more choice in what stories arise in us with painful sensations. We can then be with pain in a more curious and friendly way.

We invite you to acknowledge any stories you have about your body and the pelvic pain you experience. You might choose to write them down, to make them explicit, instead of just a vague notion in your mind. And then we invite you to consider your body as someone you've heard rumors and stories about, but whom you've never really gotten to know one-on-one. Consider the possibility that the rumors and stories aren't true. Putting the stories aside, we can practice listening to what our body has to say, and build a relationship with the cascade of sensation below the neck. Allow trust to build gradually as you practice, noticing kindly when you get distracted or overwhelmed. Your body can be a brilliant partner with your brain, not just in tackling your pelvic pain, but in all of life.

So how do you "do" this practice? Below are some basic principles and helpful tips to support you in developing this new awareness of (and relationship with) your body.

Cultivating Somatic Awareness Practice

Just notice.

Notice: Such a simple but powerful word and practice. On the most basic level, somatic awareness is simply noticing your body. What is happening in your body when…? What do you perceive when you pause to notice what's happening? That's the whole practice really: just notice.

Differentiate between thoughts, emotions and body sensations—and then focus your curiosity and awareness on the sensations.

For many of us, when we first "check in with ourselves" we notice what we're thinking, or we might identify a feeling state, like "I feel anxious," "I hurt" or "I feel pleasure". The challenge is to drop deeper and notice the sensations happening in your body, things like temperature, vibration, tension, tingling. The cumulative effect of these sensations is how our brains ultimately interpret that we're feeling "anxious" "pain" or "pleasure". But for somatic practice...

Don't attach meaning to your sensations.

Just notice. Eventually you may learn, without effort, that a certain sensation is your body communicating something we call "meaning," but for now, just notice. Being curious isn't the same as trying to figure it all out. The more you practice, the more you'll be able to perceive, which ultimately means you're getting more information from your body when it wants to communicate meaning to you. In the meantime...

Don't freak out if you don't feel much at first—your perception will build with time and practice.

We promise. All you have to do is notice.

Don't freak out if your sensations change as soon as you notice them. Just notice the changes.

The nature of all living things is to move. Even when we're still, our blood is flowing, nerves are firing. When our sensations shift it can be a reminder that we are alive. And a reminder of possibility— uncomfortable or painful sensations move eventually, as do pleasurable ones. We're not stuck. We're alive. Our attention is an energy, and often that burst of energy inspires change, actually causing sensations to shift. Every moment we engage in somatic awareness is an opportunity to experience and observe this inherent potential in all of us for change.

Build a vocabulary of sensation – literally.

It can be hard to identify what we feel if we don't have words to express it. Following is a list of words that you may find helpful when getting started with describing bodily sensations. Add to it as you dive deeper into your somatic awareness!

Figure 1: Table of Somatic Sensations[2]

Buzzing	Fluttery	Twitchy	Cold	Tingling	Flowing
Clammy	Dizzy	Floating	Hot	Fuzzy	Contained
Jagged	Tight	Prickly	Heavy	Itchy	Frozen
Dense	Liquid	Numb	Light	Constricted	Jumpy
Stabbing	Aching	Throbbing	Streaming	Hollow	Dense

---

[2] adapted from Peter Levine

There is no "right" way to feel

Particularly for those of us who struggle with perfectionism or who were socialized in religious, moral, or cultural traditions that taught us that "right and wrong" are static answers, listening to our body without judgment can be a real challenge. You are literally learning to hear your body's own truth. You are learning to trust yourself. Acknowledge how new this is and then let yourself off the hook and go back to just noticing. You don't have to "do" anything else.

Practice anywhere and all the time

What do you feel in your body in the shower? Standing in line at the grocery store? When the phone rings? Just notice. Start to say it out loud. Create conversations about sensation. When your friend tells you about a fight with their boss, ask them what they feel in their body as they tell you. Notice what sensations you feel in your body as they tell you about theirs.

Observing without judging quiets the inner monologue

Without training and practice, our "thinking brain" automatically defaults to anxious rumination. By training our brain to focus instead on "just noticing," we can quiet this inner monologue, and change our relationship with pain. Practice "just noticing" how the thinking brain wants to fix, change, get help, stop feeling difficult feelings, and find a way out of persistent pain. Then refocus on sensations.

Inner Monologue

Without Somatic Awareness	**With Somatic Awareness**
I feel the pain again	I notice stabbing sensation in my left ovary
I can't do this anymore	
The medicine isn't working	Breathing out. The sensation shifts to a dull ache across my pelvic bowl
It's taking too long	
That doctor doesn't get it	I feel a tightening in my chest
I won't be able to have sex tonight	Breathing in, I feel hot stabbing
My relationship is on the line	I notice my feet heavy on the earth
I can't go to work feeling this way	Tingling in my toes and fingers
It hurts!	My legs are warm and buzzing

Pain sensations are not static. They come and go, changing in intensity and variety with every breath. Ideas about pain and worries about the consequences of pain can become fixed and overwhelming. With attention to specific sensation within the body, plus the sensations of breathing, hearing, smelling, seeing, tasting and touching or being touched, we foster our capacity for non-judgemental awareness. We then have choice; we can pick to quiet the anxious rumination of the thinking mind when we want to.

Anxious rumination about the past and future consequences of pain can be very helpful when we need to figure out strategies and assess dangers. But it might be very unhelpful for the task of living with pain from moment-to-moment.[3]

Somatic awareness is a practice (not a perfect!) that can support us in the daily task of living with pain and discomfort of various kinds. When we can choose to "just notice" intense sensation, without judging, assessing consequences or looking for a way out, we can clear away some of the anxious reactivity that interferes with joyful living.

---

[3] For powerful exercises that help with the experience of acute pelvic pain, see Pam England and Rob Horowitz's book *Birthing From Within*, p. 213-239

Working in our Personal Learning Zone

As you begin to expand awareness of the pelvis, potential challenges may surface. By focusing on sensations, we bring them more clearly into our consciousness. This may mean that pain, which we have previously been able to ignore, suddenly gets bigger. Feeling sensation in a part of the body that has been hurt can invite a trauma memory or feeling to rise up unbidden. If difficult sensations, emotions or thoughts arise when doing exercises that foster pelvic floor awareness, know that this is normal. Please stop, or slow down and do less. This is not the kind of work that you can push yourself through. Explore this healing work while staying in your personal learning zone, in which you are challenging yourself just enough and not too much. In the learning zone you may feel uncomfortable, but you should never feel unsafe. Reach out for help as necessary. Talking with a friend, support group or counselor is a good way to manage difficult feelings. If your feelings are overwhelming or unmanageable, do get help from a therapist, and don't do these exercises outside the context of a supportive therapeutic environment.

Pelvic Anatomy

In a culture where genital pleasure is often shamed, and urination and defecation are considered embarrassing and dirty, the pelvis becomes an area shrouded in mystery. Although the pelvis is the most nerve-rich area of the human body, for many people there is a dearth of sensation in the pelvis. The abnegation of feeling creates what sexologists call "the Genital Hole". This phrase originated with A. H. Almaas who notes that people often experience the genital area as "a dark, empty hole, with no anatomical parts".[4]

Pelvic numbness and pelvic pain may sound like opposites, but, in fact, they are often closely related. Numbing that results from chronic anxiety, contraction and ignoring can, over time, create persistent pain. David Wise and Rodney Anderson developed a revolutionary treatment for pelvic pain at Stanford University Urology Department. They write:

> "We have identified a group of chronic pelvic pain syndromes that are caused by the overuse of the human instinct to protect the genitals, rectum and contents of the pelvis from injury or pain by contracting the pelvic

---

[4] p. 44

muscles. This tendency becomes exaggerated in predisposed individuals and over time results in pelvic pain and dysfunction. The state of chronic constriction creates pain-referring trigger points, reduced blood flow, and an inhospitable environment for the nerves, blood vessels and structures throughout the pelvic basin. This results in a cycle of pain, anxiety and tension…".[5]

We can educate and cultivate sensation with anatomical knowledge. Understanding and experiencing our pelvic anatomy can help undo the numbing of our neurology. It can also empower us to discern the exact locations of pelvic pain that otherwise seems generalized and overwhelming. With more anatomical information we will be more effective in our self-care and have a better vocabulary for communicating with doctors and partners.

Muscles of the Pelvic Floor

Humans' upright posture creates the need for a pelvic floor that is very strong; it must support all our abdominal organs and hold them in place. The pelvic floor also provides passages for urination, defecation and penetrative sexual activity. These passages need to open and close frequently. Sometimes the pelvic floor provides an opening large enough to birth a baby! Strong and flexible; open and supportive; mobile and stable: great elasticity is needed to contain these opposites.[6]

The pelvic floor muscles play an important role in posture and movement; they are key to the dynamic stability of our musculoskeletal structure. They also play a vital role in breathing. We can enhance pelvic floor awareness by simply noticing - or imagining - a deep breath going right down into the pelvic floor. We tend to think of breath as involving only the lungs and the thoracic

---

[5] p. 91

[6] As Eric Franklin notes in his book *Pelvic Power*.

diaphragm. In fact the pelvic floor muscles function as an additional diaphragm, especially when we breathe more deeply. The pelvic floor expands and the muscle fibers slide apart as we breathe in. The pelvic floor contracts and the muscle fibers slide together as we breathe out.

Figure 2: Breath engages the whole body, including the pelvis

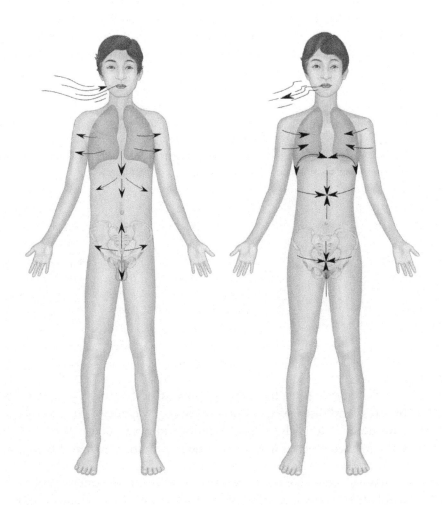

The bony structures of the pelvis are actually meant to open slightly as we breathe in and come together as we breathe out. Although this can be hard to actually feel if we are not used to attending to subtle sensations in our pelvis, we can cultivate more pelvic awareness by just imagining this process. Imagine each breath massaging and expanding the pelvic floor from the inside. Notice any sensation. Notice tension, immobility, looseness, elasticity, feelings of pain, and feelings of pleasure in the nerve-rich pelvis. If it does not exacerbate tension in your pelvis, you can occasionally gently engage the pelvic floor muscles on the out-breath, and relax those muscles on the in-breath. Engage the pelvic floor muscles that you use to stop yourself from pooing or peeing. Feel deeply into the relaxation and ease of letting go.

Figure 3: Pelvic Mobility

The bony structures of the pelvis are meant to open slightly as we breathe in and come together as we breathe out.

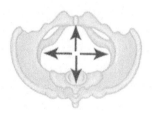 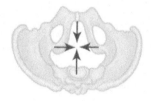

When we note that pelvic pain can be triggered or exacerbated by stress and distress, this does not in any way mean "the pain is all in your head". Our pelvic floor functions in a way that is intricately and intimately connected with our thoughts, environment and feelings.

With any increase in anxiety, our nervous system mobilizes a whole-body response. We brace for action. The pelvic floor is the core structure involved in this process. We have all seen dogs raise their tails when on alert. And we've seen them pulling their tails between their legs, indicating fearful, self-protective surrender.

Humans do something very similar with their pelvic floor muscles, despite the absence of a visible tail. If we are afraid, vigilant and on alert, there will be one kind of pelvic floor activation (tail raised). If we feel defeated, withdrawn or ashamed, there is another kind of pelvic floor activation (tail tucked in). Both involve unconscious clenching of pelvic floor muscles.

When there is a clench in our pelvic floor muscles, the flow of blood and lymph is impaired. If a pelvic clench persists, there can be consequences throughout our bodies and being. The function and flexibility of pelvic sphincters is reduced. Organs can become stuck to other organs and surrounding tissues (see the chapter on "Pelvic Scars and Fascial Adhesions"). Information flows less freely through nerves that relay sensation to and from skin and muscles, and feeling may diminish (creating areas of numbness) or get stuck on "high" (creating areas of hypersensitivity and pain), or both. Contraction, pain, numbness, inflexibility and diminished mobility and flow in our tissues comprise the physiology of chronic anxiety. This physiology supports the brain in anxious thoughts, generating more stress-based neurochemistry. A feedback loop can be created that amplifies pelvic pain from different sources.

Pelvic floor clenching is an autonomic nervous system reaction; it happens without our conscious awareness. When we bring our conscious attention to the muscles of the pelvic floor, we can open a portal to our autonomic nervous system, and create more choice in how we feel and function.

Just as chronic tension in the pelvic floor feeds anxiety and vigilance, a pelvic floor that is more flexible supports us in feeling relaxed, resilient and resourced. The simple exercise of "massaging" the pelvic floor with our inner awareness and deep breath can help us feel more spaciousness, ease and aliveness in our cells and our souls.

The muscles of the pelvic floor can also be felt and massaged by reaching inside the anus or vagina. Instructions on pelvic floor massage are included in the chapter on "Touch-based Treatment".

A note on Kegels: It is often suggested that people do exercises called "Kegels" – consciously exaggerating pelvic floor muscle tension. Kegels seem to be prescribed for everything from stopping urinary incontinence to making vaginas "tighter" (a problematic word, but that's another book perhaps). However, these exercises are not appropriate for anyone with an already contracted pelvic floor, in which case they can even create injury, pain and adhesions. Muscle fibers that are already spastic or holding profound tension cannot be engaged and strengthened by conscious squeezing. The pelvic floor has a foundational need for flexibility. Please do not practice Kegels if the muscles of your pelvic floor are tight. Once this tension is released and muscle elasticity is available, *then* it is safe to cultivate strength in the muscles of the pelvic floor.

To assess pelvic floor tension, feel into the pelvic outlet from the outside, pressing fingers deep into the area extending from between the sit bones up towards the pubic bone. You may feel tense and painful areas. You can also feel into the pelvic diaphragm from inside the vagina or anus. Using lubricant, enter and press your thumb into various areas of the pelvic floor. Some areas may feel tight or painful, while other areas feel flaccid, and other areas feel healthy and resilient. Massage, exercises like the ones described in this book, deep breathing, and bringing more ease and pleasure into your life are all important ways to ease pelvic floor tension. See more in the chapter on "Touch-based Treatment".

Figure 4: The pelvic diaphragm from above

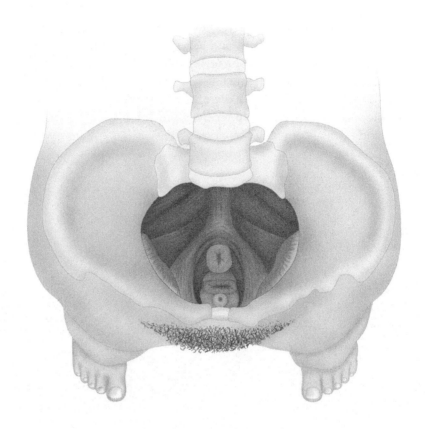

The Boney Bowl of the Pelvis

The boney bowl of the pelvis consists of the hipbones, joined at the front by the pubic bone (pubic symphysis) and at the back by the sacrum. Feel the bony landmarks. The pelvic crest, the upper boundary of your pelvic bowl, can be felt by putting your hands on each side of your hips. Move your hands to the front of your pelvis, just above your genitals, to feel where these bones join together at the pubic bone. Opposite the pubic bone, and at the back of the body, feel the sacrum. Move your hand down to the bottom of your buttocks to find the sit bones (the ischeal tuberosities). Feel into the front half of the pelvic opening by feeling from sit bone to pubic bone, on each side separately. Feel into the back part of the opening with a hand on the sacrum and a hand on the sit bone, on each side. Feel the opening from front to back by putting a hand on the pubic bone in the front and the tailbone (coccyx) at the bottom of the sacrum in the back. Our pelvic bowl can be visualized as a sacred chalice that simultaneously receives life force energy, holds it within us, and births it out into the world.

Figure 5: The boney bowl of the pelvis

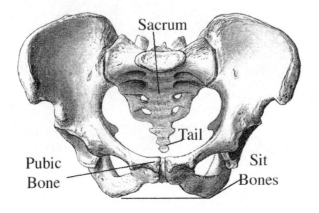

Genital Anatomy and Mapping

As somatic sex educators we know it is very common for people not to know their own genitals, nor to understand genital anatomy. It is common to be unable to describe to others what kind of touch hurts and what we like. Many people whose lives are terribly impacted by genital pain can neither discern for themselves, nor describe to medical professionals or partners, precisely where and how they are experiencing the pain. Here we offer some basic genital anatomy so that readers can begin to develop the language with which to recognize and understand their genital structures and communicate more clearly about pain and pleasure with doctors and partners.

We recommend that, rather than simply reading this anatomy material, you use these pages as a guide to "map" your own unique genitals. There are a variety of ways to explore genital mapping. A simple way to get started is to use self-touch, a mirror and the anatomy diagrams here to explore and orient to your genital landscape. Once oriented, we invite you to try different ways of touching those parts. You may wish to observe the changes in your genitals when engorged compared to unengorged. Feeling into our anatomy, learning to discern sensation in different parts of the body, and experimenting with bringing greater awareness to the way our anatomy responds to arousal and orgasm, are all part of developing our personal pain and pleasure "literacy". With this knowledge and somatic awareness, we may not only find ways to pinpoint and communicate about specific pain issues, but also find ways to work and play around them. Thus understanding our genital anatomy helps us to get the professional support we may need while creating an opportunity for us to stay connected to our pleasure and eroticism during and beyond treatment or recovery.

Genital structure, shape, size and function are hugely diverse. Just as every human face is unique, even though we share enough similarities to name the "parts" of our face—nose, mouth, eyes – so too are all of our genitals unique. In addition to externally visible variance, there are big differences in the structure and density of genital nerves, affected by pre-natal hormone levels, random chance in the timing of fetal development, life experience and many other factors.

There is also great diversity in how people want to name their genitals. Everyone has the right to self-define their genitals in ways that feel right for them. The anatomy drawings and labels here offer names for genital structures that are likely to be understood by medical professionals. When mapping our own genitals, we can find ways of naming different body parts that feel right for us. When mapping another person's genitals, we always ask about the names they prefer.

Homologous Genital Structures

In embryonic development, we all have bi-potential genital tissues. At around 7 weeks our genitals begin to differentiate to some degree in the presence or absence of a Y chromosome. The homology of genital structures persists into adult life, as can be seen in the illustration opposite. So-called male and female genitals are not so different. We all have inner bits and outer bits and beds of erectile tissue.

Understanding the basic homology of genital structures is supportive when we are feeling our way into a gender identity that is different from what someone looking at our genitals naively might suppose. It is vitally important that in mapping our genital anatomy we use and create language that resonates for us. We can self-define our genitals in ways that support our gender journey, as that evolves throughout life.

The search for support and treatment for pelvic pain becomes unimaginably more complicated for trans and gender non-binary people when the right to self-identify and the diversity of the gender galaxy are not respected or understood. Finding providers who are knowledgeable in pelvic pain conditions and treatments is challenging for everyone, but trans, non-binary and gender non-conforming people risk being mis-gendered or treated with aversion by ignorant providers, exposing themselves to additional stress or potentially traumatizing interactions. While we continue to educate and advocate within the medical community (and the world at large) to make the gender galaxy safe for all of us, we hope that the gender-inclusive, pleasure-based approach of this book can begin to make it safer for people of all genders to address pelvic pain and access pelvic pleasure.

Figure 6: Homologous Genitals

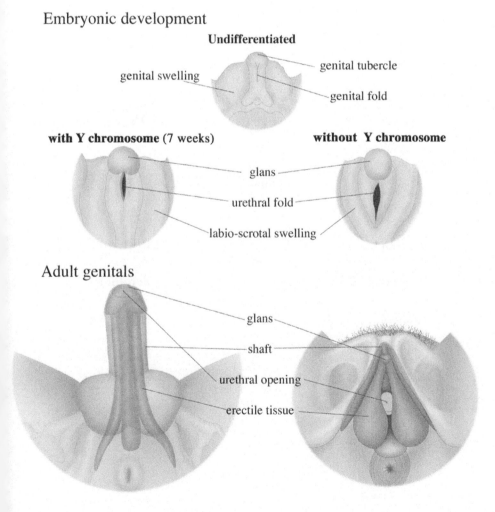

Embryonic development

Undifferentiated

genital swelling — genital tubercle

— genital fold

with Y chromosome (7 weeks)   **without Y chromosome**

glans

urethral fold

labio-scrotal swelling

Adult genitals

glans

shaft

urethral opening

erectile tissue

Genital Nerves

The pudendal nerve largely innervates the external structures of vulva and penis. Internally, the pelvic nerve provides the nerve supply of the vagina, cervix, rectum and bladder plus the deeper structures of the penis. The hypogastric nerve conveys sensory activity from the uterus and cervix and the prostate gland and testicles. The cervix and uterus are also innervated by the vagus nerve, which travels from the brain through the body outside the spinal cord.

Figure 7: Pelvic Nerves Diagrammed

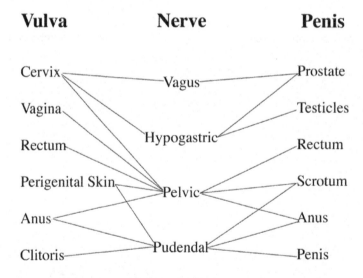

Figure 8: Pelvic Nerves Illustrated

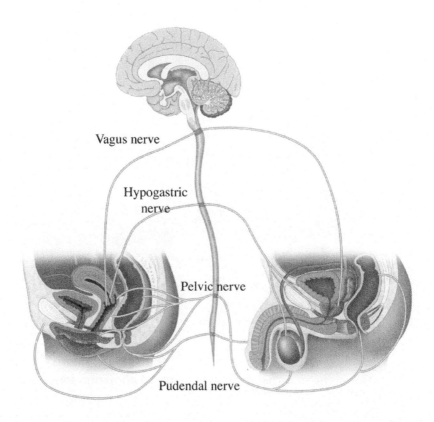

Penis Anatomy

Figure 9: Penis Anatomy, external parts

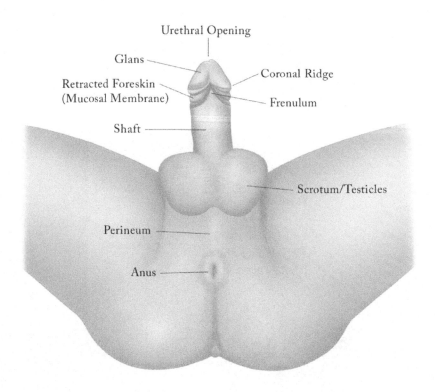

Penises come in a vast diversity of unique configurations, shapes and sizes.

The skin covering the external penis is specialized tissue, composed of skin, mucosa, nerves, blood vessels, and muscle fibers. The tissue of the foreskin has great elasticity. In adults it can stretch and roll out when the penis is erect, and afterwards return to its forward, protective position. (In young children the foreskin is fused to the glans and does not retract.) In the forward position the foreskin functions to protect the mucosal surface of the glans. The fibers of the peripenic muscle sheath form a whorl at the tip of the foreskin, which acts as a sphincter (the preputial sphincter). Inside the foreskin, the skin is moist mucosal tissue.

Up to half the penis is inside the body, and its tissues can usually be felt by reaching behind the scrotum to the perineum. The perineum and the scrotum are highly innervated and often can be very sensitive to touch. Internal anatomical structures are also highly innervated, particularly the prostate gland. The striated muscles of the pelvic floor surround, support, protect and stimulate these internal structures.

The prostate gland is wrapped around the urethra, just under the bladder. (The urethra is the tube that carries urine and ejaculate out of the body.) The prostate gland is partly muscular and partly glandular. The smooth muscle of the prostate pulses during orgasm. (Smooth muscle is innervated autonomically; we normally cannot move these muscles with our conscious mind.)

The corpus cavernosum is the anatomical name for the erectile tissues of the penis (and the clitoris). Blood vessels in this specialized tissue contain one-way valves that can close to allow engorgement, with sufficient stimulation in a relaxed environment.

Arousal and erection are not equivalent. Pleasurable arousal and orgasm can happen without any engorgement of the genital tissues. Conversely, the complex reflex responses of engorgement and ejaculation can occur without pleasure or arousal. Healthy genital tissues engorge several times during the night, in cycles related to REM sleep. Engorgement and ejaculation sometimes occur during the horror of a sexual assault.

Touch needs and preferences can also change from day to day and moment to moment. Touch sensitivity, pleasure and pain can be affected by many factors including tissue health, hormonal balance, mental focus, the degree of arousal and the stage of life.

Figure 10: Penis anatomy, saggital view

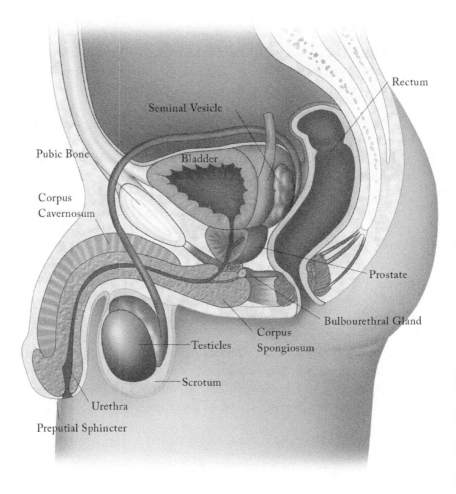

Figure 11: External penis showing possible changes with arousal and engorgement

When erectile tissues are not engorged, the foreskin completely covers the glans. As the corpus cavernosum fills with blood, the penis expands in size. The loose skin of the foreskin retracts, exposing the glans. Bulbourethral glands (aka Cowper's glands) secrete pre-cum. With the foreskin fully retracted, the mucosal membrane of the glans and inner foreskin is exposed. Urethral opening dilates, glans color deepens. Testicles elevate and rotate forward.

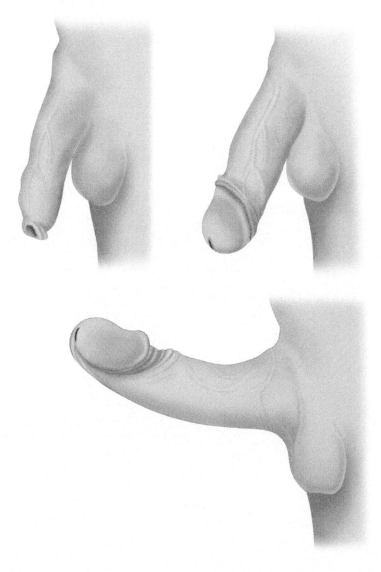

Figure 12: Cross-section of the penis, showing erectile tissue

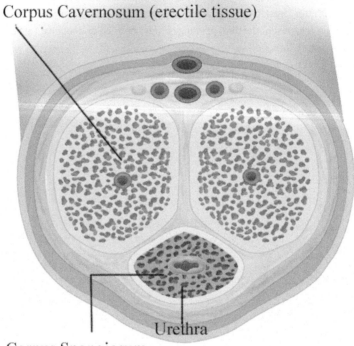

Figure 13: Circumcision Styles

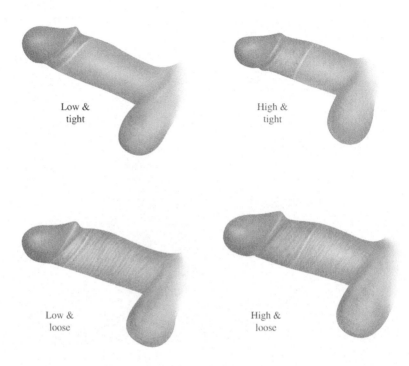

The skin can be tight on a circumcised penis, showing no mobility during erection, sometimes triggering pain during penetrative sex. (For more on circumcision mapping and healing see a free online course on Caffyn's website.) There is a ring scar on the shaft of every circumcised penis. A difference in pigmentation between the shaft skin and the exposed inner foreskin is often quite visible. The tissue of the glans and exposed inner foreskin toughens during the healing process, and it no longer feels moist, soft and wet like mucosal tissue.

Figure 14: Pelvic floor muscles

Figure: The muscles of the pelvic floor are an integral part of sexual response and orgasm. The bulbospongiosis muscles contract with arousal and contribute to erection. The pubococcygeus muscles, and others, often pulse with orgasm.

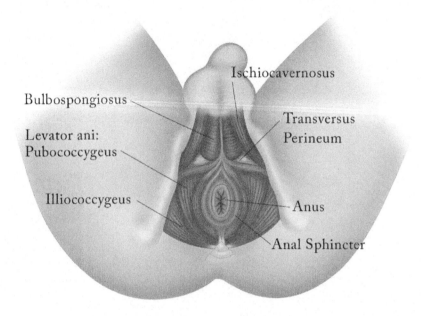

Vulva Anatomy

Figure 15: Vulva anatomy, external parts

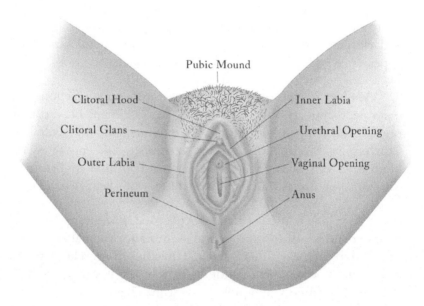

People with vulvas have their own unique anatomical configurations. Some labia are fat and some are thin. Some are long and some are short, and some are markedly asymmetrical. Sometimes the glans of the clitoris is prominent, and sometimes it seems impossibly hard to find. A huge ranges of colors, shapes and sizes all are normal and beautiful.

The inner labia meet at the center, forming a hood over the clitoral glans that protects this highly innervated area. The inside of the inner labia, and the glans, are moist mucosal tissue.

The external clitoris is actually part of a much larger clitoral complex. The erectile tissues of the clitoral complex are sandwiched between the muscles layers of the pelvic floor. Blood vessels in these tissues contain one-way valves that can close to allow engorgement, with sufficient stimulation, focused attention and a relaxed environment. There is as much erectile tissue in a vulva as in a penis, but most of it is hidden beneath the skin.

Possible changes in the external vulva with arousal and engorgement include: the clitoris may increase in size 2-3 times and protrude from beneath the hood. Outer lips become puffy, separated and elevated. Inner lips increase in size and extend outwards. The appearance and behavior of vulvas varies widely.

As for people with penises, arousal and erection are not equivalent. For people with vulvas too, pleasurable arousal and orgasm can happen without any engorgement of the genital tissues. Conversely, the complex reflex responses of engorgement and lubrication can occur without pleasure or arousal. Lubrication and orgasm sometimes occur during the horror of a sexual assault.

The vagina consists of a soft, collapsed, fibromuscular tube with an inner surface of moist mucosal membrane. Vaginal secretions can further lubricate the inner vagina. The smooth muscle of the vagina can contract when penetration is unwanted; it can expand during arousal or childbirth, and pulse at orgasm. The striated muscles of the pelvic floor also surround, support, protect and stimulate the vagina. The introitus or vaginal entry is a common location for genital pain as the skin here is relatively thin and can develop fissures. A vaginal corona — generally known as the hymen but renamed in 2009 by a Swedish sexual rights group in an attempt to dispel many of the myths surrounding hymens — is made up of thin, elastic folds of mucous membrane located just inside the entrance to the vagina. This structure or remnants of it may be visible at the introitus.

The so-called G-Spot is misnamed because it is not a single "spot". It is a cone of erectile tissue that surrounds the urethra. Different people have different urethral sponge shapes and different areas of maximum sensitivity. The glandular tissue of the G-Spot can be found on the top (anterior) wall of the vagina, beginning just inside. The tissue might have a ridged feeling. It may become more visible at the vaginal entrance with arousal and engorgement.

The internal organs are involved in sexual response. In higher states of arousal, pelvic ligaments contract, raising the uterus up over the bladder and expanding the vaginal canal.

Touch needs and preferences change from day to day and moment to moment. Touch sensitivity, pleasure and pain can be affected by many factors including tissue health, hormonal balance, mental focus, the degree of arousal and the stage of life.

Figure 16: Vulva anatomy, saggital view

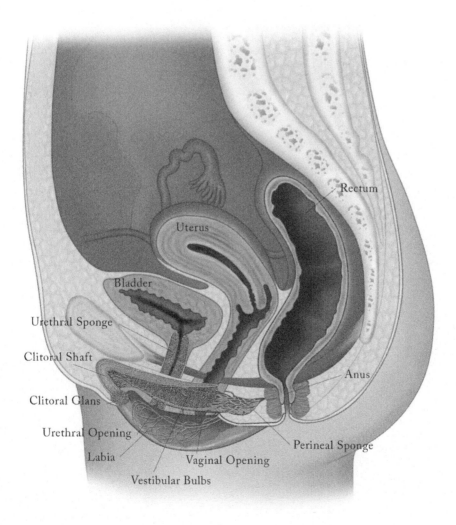

Figure 17: The erectile tissue of the vulva, unengorged and engorged

Erectile tissues of the clitoral complex become engorged with blood, including the shaft and legs of the clitoris and the vestibular bulbs.

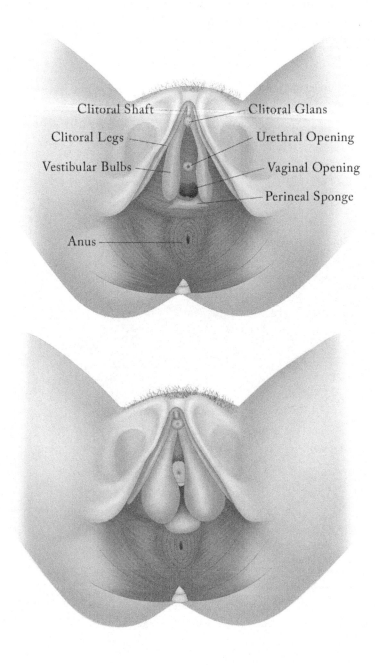

Figure 18: Possible changes to the external vulva with arousal and engorgement.

The clitoral glans may increase in size and protrude from beneath the hood. Outer lips become puffy, separated and elevated. The urethral sponge (G-Spot) may become more visible at the vaginal opening.

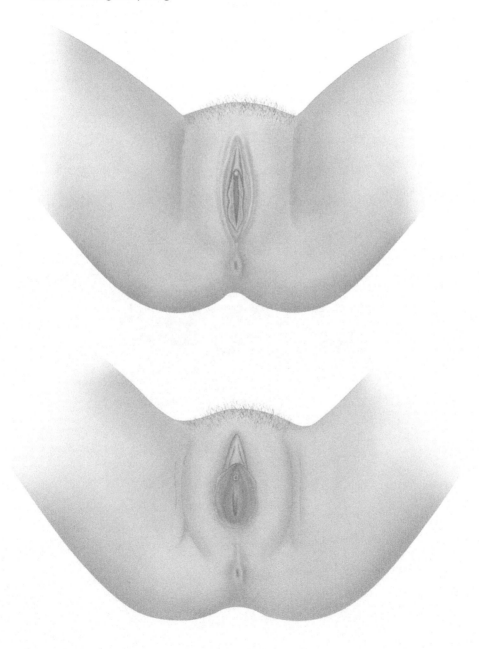

Figure 19: Muscles of the pelvic floor

These muscles are an integral part of sexual response and orgasm. The bulbospongiosis muscles contract with arousal and contribute to erection. The pubococcygeus muscles, and others, often pulse with orgasm.

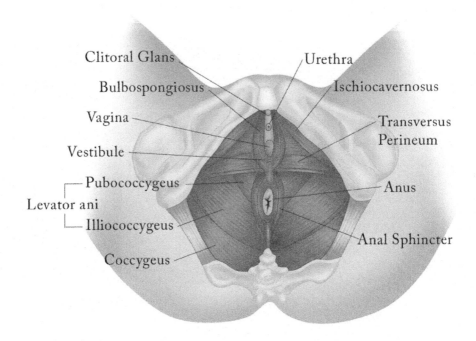

Anal Anatomy

There are two muscle rings called sphincters around the anal opening. if you insert a finger about one half-inch into the anus and press your fingertip against the side, you can feel the place where external and internal sphincter muscles overlap. We can squeeze the muscles of the external sphincter tight by an act of conscious will, just like we can purse our lips or clench a fist. The internal sphincter is quite different. This is smooth muscle controlled by the autonomic nervous system. When both of the anal sphincters are deeply relaxed, the anal opening can widen greatly. Forcing penetration without this deep relaxation can result in a variety of medical problems such as hemorrhoids (protrusion of veins from the anal cushions) or fissures (tears or cracks in the anal lining). When touch is prematurely or forcibly introduced into the anus, the sphincter muscles can go into spasm. This can also trigger spasms in other muscles of the pelvic floor.

Figure 20: Anal sphincters

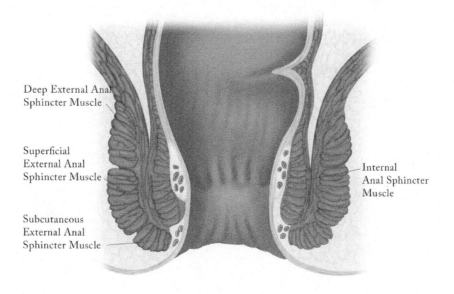

Deep External Anal Sphincter Muscle

Superficial External Anal Sphincter Muscle

Subcutaneous External Anal Sphincter Muscle

Internal Anal Sphincter Muscle

Describing Pain and Pleasure: Layers

Anatomically, there are many layers pelvic pain can stem from or be felt in:

- skin

- mucous membrane

- nerves

- scars

- adhesions

- all the striated pelvic floor muscles, or one

- smooth muscle

- bones

- joints

- organs (bladder, bowel, uterus, prostate, vagina)

- erectile tissues

- systemic (whole body functions)

Causes of Pelvic Pain

Pelvic Scars and Fascial Adhesions

A number of factors can create or contribute to pelvic pain. Often several factors exist in the body for years without causing symptoms until some event, seemingly innocuous, tips the scales into pain. In this section we discuss some frequent contributors to pelvic pain conditions. Each of these factors may provide insight into the origin of pain that is not explicable or treatable through differential medical diagnoses. This may also provide insight into ways to work with, treat, and possibly ameliorate or resolve a variety of painful conditions.

Pelvic pain is often caused or complicated by scar tissue or other adhesions in the pelvis or abdomen. To understand how this works – which will help you understand how somatic sex educators work to address these issues – let's start with some basic definitions.

Fascia is a form of connective tissue found *everywhere* in the body. It wraps around each individual muscle fiber, then wraps around the bundles of fibers, then wraps around all the bundles that form the muscle itself. It surrounds the organs and fills the space between the organs. It's like a full-body web in which all the other parts—veins, nerves, organs—are embedded. And while "web" is a great visual image, this web is dynamic, not static. The strands of the web are tiny tubules that slide easily along each other in three dimensions, constantly shifting in structure and design to allow our bodies to move, to absorb the shock of our movements and to keep nutrients, electrical impulses, fluids and neural messages flowing throughout the body. Picture them a bit like strands of egg white stretching between your fingertips. Healthy fascia is truly fluid—full of fluid and in constant fluid motion.

The egg-white–like part of fascia is called the ground substance. Within the ground substance are two other key components of fascial tissue: collagen and elastin. Collagen is a strong, dense protein, but it's not flexible. Elastin is a highly elastic, or stretchy, protein, but it's not very strong. Together these three components work to keep the body strong, flexible, and fluid.

Scars form when the integrity of body tissues are compromised - be they cut, torn, burned, or eroded (as in a sore on the skin's surface). To heal this rupture in the tissue, the body lays down collagen, that strong connective protein, to fill in the gap or knit the tissue back together. Healthy tissue also contains collagen, laid out in neat, orderly patterns that allow the tissue to move easily. The collagen in a scar is arranged randomly, like a dense birds nest pattern, making it even less flexible than tidy collagen, and susceptible to "sticking" to adjacent tissues.

When adjacent tissues stick to each other, this is called an adhesion. Tissues can adhere together because of scars, as described above, or in the presence of inflammation, chronic tension, and other injuries. Remember that fascial tissue is designed to constantly slide and glide and reorganize. When layers of tissue stick together in a scar or adhesion, our fascial web is no longer dynamic.

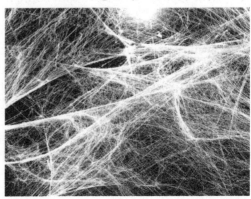

Figure 21: Image of fascia

Figure 22: Figure showing (a) healthy muscle, (b) response to injury, and (c) fascial organization in chronic pain conditions

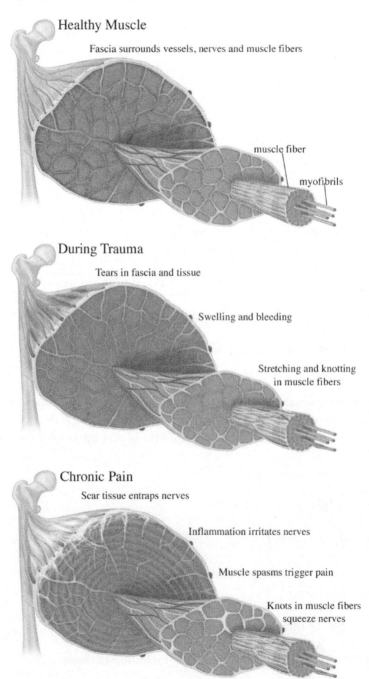

These places of dense collagen in the body compromise the fluid flexibility of the fascial web, interrupting the flow of fluids and energy impulses through the body and restricting the movement of those dynamic tubules of the ground substance. Fascial fibers begin to stick together and dehydrate. This lack of movement and health in one place in the body spreads strain throughout the body, often in wide and unpredictable patterns. Imagine that your fascial web is like a sweater; as you pull one corner of the sweater, you can see the stress of that pull on the individual stitches and the weave of the sweater as a whole. Scars and adhesions pull on your fascia in the same way. Your body adjusts to accommodate to this strain, but over time the stress of the pull causes inflammation and adhesions in other parts of your body. In this way scars beget more scars. Tension begets more tension. Often this is when pain symptoms begin – perhaps years after the original injury, and with the pain not manifesting at the site of the originally compromised tissue.

Scars and adhesions in the pelvis can be caused by:

- Abdominal surgeries of all kinds

- Episiotomy, tearing, or general tissue trauma during childbirth

- Inflammation from infections such as sexually transmitted infections, bladder infections, urinary tract infections, or any of the many conditions that cause bowel inflammation

- Endometriosis

- Falling on your tailbone

- Radiation treatment

- Postural misalignment resulting in compression of pelvic structures

- Tissue trauma during rape or sexual assault

- Genital surgeries of all kinds, including labioplasty,

circumcision, cliterodectomy

- Gender confirmation surgeries

- Tissue trauma from engaging in consensual penetrative sex without adequate arousal or lubrication

- Chronic pelvic tension

The National Institutes of Health reports that "Of patients who undergo abdominal surgery, 93% of patients develop abdominal adhesions. Surgeries in the lower abdomen and pelvis, including bowel and gynecological operations, carry an even greater chance of abdominal adhesions. Abdominal adhesions can become larger and tighter as time passes, sometimes causing problems years after surgery".[7] They comment, incorrectly, that "Surgery is the only way to treat abdominal adhesions that cause pain, intestinal obstruction, or fertility problems" while noting that additional surgery "carries the risk of additional abdominal adhesions". As this book goes to press, statistics show that over 30% of people who give birth in the US have a cesarean delivery (up from 5% in 1970), and yet there is little to no information provided about tending to scars and abdominal adhesions during the postpartum period. See chapters in this book on Touch-based Treatment and Topical Treatments for safer, natural options for addressing abdominal adhesions.

---

[7] National Institute of Diabetes and Digestive and Kidney Diseases

Figure 23: Pelvic adhesions

Adhesions
extend into the
abdomen, affecting
digestion and
other functions

The colon can adhere
to the posterior wall of
the uterus
Ovaries may adhere
to pelvic
ligaments

Adhesions from
vaginal scarring affect
sexual function and
urinary function

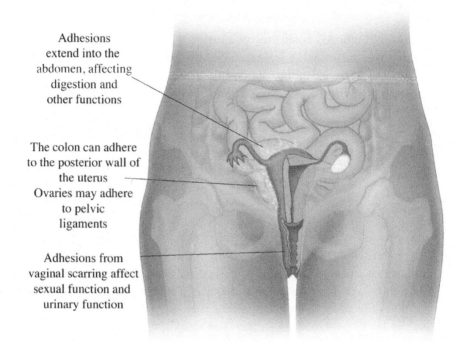

Pelvic Pain and Trauma

High rates of sexual and physical abuse and other traumas have consistently been shown in studies of people with persistent pelvic pain. Having a trauma-aware practice is vital for health-care practitioners in this field. Feeling empowered to work with our own traumas effectively is an important aspect of addressing pelvic pain.

There are many varieties of trauma. Trauma can mean a single big event such as a rape or assault, or involve ongoing experiences of abuse, shame, bullying, or sexual violence. Violence also happens in ways that affect whole groups and communities, through systemic oppressions, historic inequities, gender-based and racialized violence. Gender norms are enforced with violence as part of a traumatic acculturation around sex.

We live in a society where sexual violence is ubiquitous. Yet we observe that some people are resilient; the trauma they experience does not seem to affect their pelvic floor health, or have a deep and lasting impact on their lives and relationships. Trauma affects different people quite differently. As Peter Levine observes, "Trauma is in the nervous system, not in the event". Some people are resourced with resilient nervous systems; they can shake off trauma. For others, a complex and individual mix of heredity, environment and experience makes their nervous systems more vulnerable, and trauma has profound and lasting effects.

Trauma is experienced biophysically whenever the events of our lives overwhelm our ability to cope. Stress and trauma are physiologically related; cumulative stress can also overwhelm and damage the nervous system. Studies show that neglect has neurological effects that are damaging in ways very similar to violence. The nervous system can be overwhelmed by a single terrifying assault or by 1000 almost-undefinable micro-traumas. Whatever our unique story, we can trust that when we feel overwhelmed, there are biophysical consequences that are likely to have an impact on the experience of pelvic pain.

There are higher levels of cortisol and adrenaline in the blood of people with unresolved trauma. Agitation, anxiety or a sense of defeat show up in heart rate, breathing patterns, posture, tone of voice, and chronic pelvic clench. The brain's danger sensors - the amygdalae - actually become larger, and hypersensitized to danger. Stress-induced hippocampal damage affects learning and memory. Decreased medial prefrontal/anterior cingulate function means a reduced capacity for awareness, combined with a busy mind, full of intrusive or obsessive thoughts. Mechanisms that are supposed to shut off distress signals stop working (the Hypothalamus- Pituitary-Adrenal axis).

With unresolved trauma, the nervous system can be stuck on high - so that people feel continually fearful and vigilant. Or it can be stuck on low - so that people feel unalive and dissociated. Or the nervous system might cycle unpredictably between hyperarousal (anxious, distressed) and hypoarousal (numb, flat), with profound and cumulative effects on body, mind and relationships. All of these feeling states show up in the pelvic floor, which clenches when we are either anxious or discouraged.

Despite the profound consequences of unresolved trauma, we *can* foster resilience and heal the impact of trauma on our biophysical and psychosocial well-being. Somatic sex education offers specific methods for addressing trauma's imprints - see Caffyn's book *Science for Sexual Happiness*. Shauna offers Tension and Trauma Releasing Exercises (TRE®) as part of her practice. TRE® is a series of exercises that activate the body's reflex mechanism of shaking or vibrating to release trauma's imprint and bring the nervous system back to equilibrium. These exercises were originally created by Dr. David Berceli to address mass trauma in communities at war. They are now taught around the world to address not just shock trauma, but also the impacts of chronic stress endemic in modern urban life.

In addition to the specific approaches to unwinding trauma in the body that are offered by various health care practitioners, any one of us can foster our own resilience and help to undo the effects of trauma by paying attention to body sensation, tuning in to what is truly pleasurable for us, and choosing pleasure in small ways in our daily lives. See the chapters on "Befriending the Body" and "Beyond Pain to Pleasure" to learn more about cultivating these practices. In each of us, there is a biological impulse to "homeostasis" – a state of dynamic stability and maximum wellness. This inner impulse to wellbeing can always guide us to full thriving, if we give it our attention and respect.

When addressing and releasing the biophysical effects of trauma, it is always important to avoid damaging and retraumatizing. Bessel van der Kolk cautions, "For our physiology to calm down, heal and grow we need a visceral feeling of safety". The imprint of trauma on the nervous system often means that we feel chronically unsafe. We are impaired in our ability to track our needs in the moment, and to communicate well with health care providers and partners.

A trauma-informed approach to pelvic pain will emphasize the safety of the person receiving treatment. Rather than *assuming* that people have agency, choice and power in their relationship with health care providers, trauma-aware practitioners understand that safety and choice are built by acts, attitudes and experiences that foster trust. This means slowing down enough for clients to attend to their feelings and guide their experience, without pressure to move from A to Z in a given time frame. Understanding the effects of trauma, practitioners can also track and notice when people become frightened, hyperactivated, frozen, checked out or dissociated. Willingness to stop, check in, and wait for a client to be able to communicate what is going on will help avoid the dangers of retraumatization. Trauma-aware practitioners build empowering collaborative relationships that emphasize their clients' choice and agency, rather than promoting the idea that people get fixed with a practitioner's expert knowledge.

Caffyn has had the opportunity to work with many different health care practitioners over three decades of addressing persistent pelvic pain. They were especially thrilled when they had the opportunity to receive assessment and treatment for genital pain at an esteemed Vulvodynia Clinic. All went well until the physical exam, when the doctor's too-quick touch triggered an acute episode of genital pain that lasted months. Hurting instead of helping was the last thing this caring doctor intended. Caffyn "knew" cognitively that the doctor was safe. They wanted the exam, but their body reacted based on the cellular imprint of past trauma. This unfortunate dynamic could have been avoided if exam protocols had involved the patient guiding the healthcare practitioner's touch, both verbally and manually. Furthermore, to be trauma-informed there must be time enough to go slowly, without any sense of necessity to accomplish a specific physical exam at a given appointment. There must be awareness of the difficulty any trauma survivor will have in guiding someone's touch, and there must be a commitment to allowing a patient-directed process to unfold in its own time.

Bringing trauma awareness into intimate relationships is just as important. Slowing down sexual interactions, removing agendas for specific forms of sex, and living a commitment to fostering trust and empowered communication, rather than assuming it, are all vital for establishing safe-enough intimate relationships to support resilience and allow healing. It is commonplace for people to experience retraumatization to genital tissues with every sexual encounter or medical exam, without ever communicating about their pain to partners or health care practitioners.

Embodied Sex Negativity and Pelvic Pain

While it's vital to talk about trauma, both as a cause of and a consideration during treatment of pelvic pain, what about people who haven't experienced trauma and yet live with chronic pelvic pain? You might be asking, "Why am I in experiencing a chronic pelvic clench or a sense of being overwhelmed if I've never experienced a traumatic event?"

Pelvic pain can sometimes emerge as a result of negative messages we receive about sex. [8] If you were taught that sex is bad or dangerous, your body may have internalized those messages. If you received inadequate sex education, perhaps suggesting that sex is always painful or that you will always be at risk for pregnancy or sexually transmitted infections, your body may be armoured against sex. So now when you begin to engage sexually with a partner or yourself, or perhaps simply attempt to insert a tampon, your body contracts, clenching your pelvic floor and the smooth muscles of the pelvis to protect you in a dangerous situation. That protective contraction could make penetrative sex painful. Or, for some people, the contraction is so intense that penetration of any kind is impossible. In people with vaginas this situation is usually diagnosed as vaginismus. One client with vaginismus reported that when her partner attempted to insert his penis in her vagina, he said it felt like he "hit a brick wall".

---

[8] This chapter is inspired by M. and L. Carter's writing on overcoming vaginismus as well as our work with clients.

Perhaps you're thinking, "But I don't think sex is bad now! I don't believe all those things I was told as a kid. I *want* to have intercourse with my partner. So why is this still happening?" Remember that your body is it's own wondrous intelligence, as well as a record of all you've experienced and been taught. For how many years were you bombarded with these messages or indoctrinated with these beliefs? And how implicitly did your young self trust that the adults who told you this were infallible and had your best interest at heart? Your mind may have a new idea about sex, but your body spent years believing that sex was bad or dangerous and that you must be protected. Your nervous system is now responding with the same hypervigilance as a person who has experienced an identifiable shock trauma. And like all nervous system trauma responses, it is not consciously controlled. A person experiencing these contractions is not "making them happen" and can't just "make it stop". It will take time and patient practice to discharge the imprint those old beliefs have left on the body, and to get the body and the mind on the same page about sex and safety. All the resources and techniques recommended for shock trauma apply to resolving the impact of these embodied sex-negative beliefs as well.

Sometimes there is no identifiable cause, physical or non-physical, of pelvic pain. Luckily, when we work directly with the body, we don't need to know the cause of our pain to work with it and through it. Whether or not you identify as a survivor of trauma, whether or not you can identify a physical, psychological or emotional "cause" of your pelvic pain, it is still possible to relieve pain and find more pleasure in the pelvis.

Treatments

Touch-based Treatment

Precautions and Possibilities with Touch

Trauma survivors with distressed nervous systems often recoil from touch and may experience all touch as assaultive. But once the capacity for empowered choice and voice is built, and touch is requested and directed by clients at a pace that is slow enough to avoid triggering nervous system distress, then touch itself has many profound biophysical effects that can support recovery. Touch shifts our neurochemical environment so we can feel more relaxation and connection. Touch brings us into our bodies, supporting us in consciously following our pleasure rather than unconsciously shrinking from our pain. Touch encourages the circulation of blood and lymphatic fluid, and fascial release. It supports the softening and distensibility of tissues for health and healing. Trauma expert Bessel van der Kolk writes, "Given the subcortical nature of trauma imprints, effective therapy needs to help survivors tolerate the sensory reminders of the trauma, and physically experience efficacy and purpose in response to stimuli that once triggered feelings of helplessness and dependence".[9]

Working with the Fascia in the Pelvis

The instructions here can be for self-administered touch or for receiving touch from a partner or professional practitioner. (Somatic sex educators are trained to offer myofascial release-based work for pelvic pain as well as genital massage and pleasure coaching.) Whether administered by a somatic sex educator, a partner, or yourself, the "how to" principles of touch for transforming pelvic pain are the same. We approach persistent pelvic pain through the lens of myofascial release techniques. Other terms you may hear are "pelvic release" or "genital dearmouring". This is a different approach from what is typically thought of as massage, where the tissue is stroked, kneaded or plucked.

In traditional massage, the hands administering touch are dynamic, moving and "working with" the tissue. This kind of massage, when it includes the genitals, is often helpful for creating a new approach to pelvic sensation, supporting warm erotic connection in the presence of persistent genital pain, and allowing for a non-demand and trauma-informed approach to engaging with erotic energy. For more on this see Caffyn's book *Erotic Massage*.

The myofascial release techniques that we explain in this chapter differ from traditional massage techniques. In myofascial release-based touch, the hands administering touch apply gentle pressure to the affected tissue, feeling into the extent of the tissue's flexibility, which is often referred to as "the resilient edge of resistance".[10] Under this gentle pressure, the tissue itself begins to unwind, to melt, to become unstuck and rehydrated. The hands of the person providing touch move only when the tissue underneath their fingers moves, and they follow the lead of the healing body.

---

[9] van der Kolk, 2002

[10] This phrase originated with Chester Mainard.

How is this possible? Remember our introduction to fascia in the chapter on "Pelvic Scars and Fascial Adhesions". The gelatinous nature of the ground substance responds to the heat of the provider's hands, literally softening or melting. As the tissue softens, fluid can return to the previously collapsed tubules, bringing fluidity and mobility back to the tissue. It is also theorized that since the living fascia has a crystalline structure, the mechanical pressure applied by the provider's hands creates an electric polarization in the fascia, changing the structure of the tissue. This is a phenomenon known as piezoelectricity. As the tissue begins to restructure, the provider of touch gently follows the movement of the tissue with their fingers or hands, until the tissue completes its reorganization and becomes still. It usually takes 30-90 seconds for the tissue to begin to respond, and often 3-5 minutes of movement before the tissue re-stabilizes. This is a very slow, very gentle form of touch.

Your pain will guide you as you apply touch. Gently apply pressure to the painful places, with just-enough pressure to contact the tissue. Imagine the weight of a nickel—that's the right amount of pressure to apply. Stay with your body as you receive this touch; if at any point you notice you are "bracing", contracting muscles anywhere in your body to manage or endure the pain, stop and back off. Creating more contraction in the body is counterproductive. You should not apply pressure directly to a painful location if the pain is so great that your body braces. Breathe and bring awareness to exactly where the touch is placed. If you find yourself checking out, pause or go slower. Explore touch in areas around the painful spot— can you find a place where you can receive touch, stay completely relaxed, and observe what is happening in your body? Fascia is a continuous web throughout your entire organism. The release that begins in a less painful place ultimately connects to the places of your greatest pain. Trust the body to unwind in its own time.

Begin myofascial release on the external abdomen. If you are able to administer self-touch or you have access to a trusted touch provider, include the whole pelvis, and eventually, the external genitals. If the body wants internal work, these principles of myofascial release can be applied to work within the vagina and the anus. Internal touch allows access to the vast networks of fascia that support and separate the organs within the pelvic bowl.

Observing your sensation as you receive this form of touch is an incredible opportunity to expand your somatic awareness as you feel the tissue move and reorganize in your body. You may actually feel a sensation of the tissue physically moving within you. You may feel a "melting" sensation or a burning sensation, which is normal and common as fascia releases. You may feel heat in the tissue, which is a normal discharge process. As long as you are not bracing into or contracting with these sensations, just keep noticing and enjoy witnessing your body begin to heal itself. If at any point the sensations are overwhelming, frightening or too painful, stop the touch immediately.

Instead of noticing all these challenging and interesting sensations, you may simply feel numbness. This is also very normal. By attending to the numbness with kindness and acceptance, you invite it to unwind and transform. Often it can help to *imagine* the tissue melting, even visualizing a pat of butter melting in a pan or on hot toast. With time, you'll likely begin to notice sensation and change.

Notice also if you become aware of sensations in other parts of your body, parts not "directly" connected to the area being touched. Because fascia is a continuous web, those places are, in fact, connected, which is what that sensation conveys. This kind of feedback can be used to direct future touch when appropriate. For example, if as gentle pressure is applied to the upper left quadrant of the vagina, sensation is felt in the perineum, so gentle pressure can next be applied to the perineum. (Rest a gently closed fist against the perineum and apply gentle pressure in toward the body.) Think of this as the body asking for what touch it wants or needs next. From gentle pressure in the lower right quadrant of the anus, we may feel sensation in the shoulder. Feel into the connection between the anus and the shoulder, and find a touch that would support expansion and unwinding.

Another great way to direct your exploration of this kind of release in the pelvis is to apply an internal mapping approach. Imaging the vagina or anus is the face of a clock. Once you've guided your partner or practitioner's finger into the vagina or anus, apply gentle pressure at 12 o'clock. What do you notice? Is there is a sense of tightness or pain here? Stay with the tissue utilizing the basic principles described above until it ceases to unwind. Then move onto 1—what do you notice? The amount of gentle pressure that feels right will vary at each hour. Pressure at 12 and 6 o'clock on the urethral and perineal sponges can be irritating unless someone is engorged. Follow the unwinding of the tissue as above. Move onto 2 on our imaginary clock. This same pattern can be repeated at various hours and different depths of insertion in both the anus and vagina.

Figure 24: Consider the opening of the vagina or anus like the face of a clock

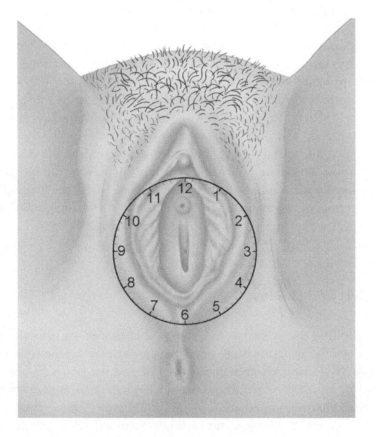

A range of emotions can accompany this unwinding practice: grief, rage, fear, gladness, power. Pleasure and pain often coexist in intricate patterns. Personal, cultural and ancestral stories often surface when working with the fascia in this way. It is important to receive touch from someone who is willing and able to hear these stories as they arise.

As previously mentioned, you can apply these principles when administering self-release. How is that physiologically possible? For some people, it may be accessible and comfortable to apply these release techniques with their own hands. For others, sex toys can be used to reach and apply gentle pressure to tense tissues. In particular, Shauna recommends the Pure Wand by njoy or The Original Crystal Wand by Nectar Products. These toys are designed and marketed for G-spot or prostate stimulation. They are curved in such a way as to allow access to and leverage on targeted areas in the anus or vagina. Any similarly shaped product will work in much the same way if you already have a toy with this shape in your toy chest. Experiment with ways to position your body to find the most comfortable way to work with your own tissue. Possible positions include: laying on your back (perhaps with a pillow under your pelvis), laying on your side (adjusting your top leg as necessary for access and comfort), standing in the shower, or resting on your forearms and knees.

The Pelvis and the Jaw

In addition to working to release the tissues of the pelvis directly, consider using massage or myofascial release on the muscles of the jaw. The connection between the jaw and the pelvis has been observed by a variety of healthcare providers ranging from dentists to midwives. Michele Forsberg, a physiotherapist practicing in Colorado, writes, "Countless times while working with my pelvic dysfunction patients, I have witnessed that while releasing their fascial restrictions vaginally, the patient's jaw will be moving ever so slightly from side to side, presumably shifting to find its new home to mirror its counterpart". Ina May Gaskin, a Certified Professional

Midwife who has delivered more than 1200 babies since 1971, teaches the "sphincter law", which states that if the jaw and mouth are relaxed, the pelvis will also relax.[11] The implications of this principle during childbirth are obvious. In addition to the lived experiences of these professionals, researchers from the Hanover Medical School in Germany conducted a study in 2009 that demonstrated that myofascial release of the temporomandibular joint significantly increased the range of motion in the hip joints and that clenching the jaw reduced hip mobility.[12]

Approaching muscular tension and release from a variety of angles—literally—is generally supportive of our healing goals. In addition, the option of treating the jaw can provide a way to start experiencing some pelvic release for those who are not comfortable or able to work with their pelvis and genitals directly for any reason. Maybe the pain is too bad this week. Maybe you're triggered and until your nervous system returns to balance, your pelvis is a no-go zone. Whatever the reason, working with the jaw provides a way to continue to take ownership of your healing and support the body in releasing the tension held in the pelvis.

Using the principles of myofascial release, palpate the muscles around the jaw until you find a spot that is tight or tender. Apply pressure to this area using your finger or fingers and hold for 3-5 minutes, allowing the release to occur. Another simple, effective exercise to address jaw tension is the cork stretch. Take a wine cork and place it between your front teeth, gently biting down on it. You may have to place it the short way initially, as you want to *gently* stretch the muscles without overstretching them in any way. As your jaw releases over time, you may acquire the flexibility to place the cork the long way between your front teeth. Don't clamp down on the cork; just bite firmly enough to hold the cork in place. Hold the cork in place for 3-5 minutes or up to 10 minutes if that is pleasurable. Remove the cork and put it in a handy place so you can do this exercise again tomorrow!

---

[11] cited by Nicole Cutler

[12] Fischer et.al.

If the cork on its side doesn't feel like enough of a stretch, but the cork at its full length feels like too much, you can replace the cork with a washcloth. Roll the cloth so as to create what feels like the ideal thickness for the right amount of stretch, bend the cloth into a U-shape, and place it in your mouth with the base of the U towards your throat, wedging the cloth between your back teeth. Gently bite down as with the cork. A dry washcloth might cause a dry mouth and become uncomfortable, so dampen the cloth before putting it between your teeth. Again, gently hold here for 3-5 minutes to allow the release to occur. Repeat daily or as often as is pleasureable.

Topical Treatments

When pelvic pain results from or increases with penetrative sex, bioavailable hormones and cannabis cream can help. Anesthetic creams that numb the genitals are often recommended by medical professionals. But numbing these tissues increases the risk of additional injury. As somatic sex educators we oppose the use of anesthetic creams. We support practices that bring presence, awareness, ease and pleasure to our genitals, rather than numbing them out. We teach many joyful alternatives to penetrative sex. In addition, we suggest exploration of various topical treatments that can be effective, for some, in supporting genital tissues to become more flexible, distensible, and less painful to touch.

Bioavailable hormones

Tissue health can be supported with topical treatments that deliver bioavailable hormones. These treatments must be prescribed by a medical doctor. Caffyn has had success with estradiol mixed in organic coconut oil applied to the vaginal opening and inner labia. We suggest organic coconut oil as a more appropriate vehicle for delivering the hormone than standard emollient creams. Coconut oil is usually well-tolerated by genital tissues. (This is not true for all people. Test first, and discuss options with your pharmacist.) Suppositories can be used intervaginally to support tissue health within the vagina as well. A suppository can be created with estradiol, or a mix of estradiol and testosterone. A doctor will need to suggest an appropriate prescription for your particular condition. A compounding pharmacy can create a cream for external use, suppositories for internal use, or both, with a ratio of .01% to .05% of one or both of these hormones.

For those who are unable or unwilling to explore prescription medication, you can confer with a natural health care practitioner about Wild Yam Cream and other natural alternatives. Be sure to look for topical treatments that are liable to be well-tolerated by delicate genital tissues. Avoid perfumes and other additives that are likely to irritate and inflame.

Cannabis-infused coconut oil

Cannabis products, while not available everywhere due to legal and political reasons, can benefit pain conditions and enhance pleasure. Cannabis-infused coconut oil is a topical treatment that has been helpful to Caffyn personally, and it has also helped her in supporting clients who want to explore penetrative pleasures in the presence of pelvic pain. People report different effects with the treatment. For some, it seems to make orgasms stronger and more easily accessible. Others report finding pain relief, sometimes with an enhanced sense of being able to relax and open to pleasure. For others, there is no discernible effect. In research with cannabis, the herb has been found to reduce inflammation and pain. It can have anti-spasmodic effects on muscles and euphoric effects on mood. If you do decide to experiment with a topical cannabis cream, be sure to choose a product without additives, chemicals, or perfumes. As cannabis can have an analgesic effect, be cautious about touch once it has been applied. If your pain is not there to protect you, are you welcoming touch that might actually be harmful to delicate genital tissues? Go very slowly, notice how you feel the next day, and experiment with effects over time.

Castor Oil Packs

Castor oil is a viscous oil derived from the castor bean. While castor oil has been designated by the US Food and Drug Administration as "generally recognized as safe and effective" (GRASE) when ingested, primarily to treat constipation, we recommend its use topically, administered as a castor oil pack, to dissolve abdominal adhesions. Castor oil can also be used directly on scars on the perineum. Evidence of the medicinal use of castor oil goes back millennia; castor beans have been discovered in Egyptian tombs, and Ayurvedic healing records document their use since 2000 BC.

How castor oil works is still a bit of a mystery. Some theorize that it affects the lymphatic system, increasing the quantity of lymph and causing lymphatic vessels to contract. A small study published in the Journal of Naturopathic Medicine in 1999 documented that castor oil packs produced a "significant" temporary increase in the number of T-11 immune cells.[13] The increase peaked 7 hours after the treatment, returning to normal levels within 24 hours. These cells, a type of white blood cell, actively defend the health of the body by forming antibodies against pathogens and their toxins. A study published in 2000 in "Mediators of Inflammation," a peer-reviewed open access medical journal, documented that the main component of castor oil, ricinoleic acid (RA), exerts "remarkable analgesic and anti-inflammatory effects" when applied topically.[14]

Before using a castor oil pack, test your skin to ensure that you are not allergic to castor oil. Use a cotton swab to apply a small amount of castor oil to your inner wrist and your inner elbow. Apply a small waterproof bandage over both areas. Leave the bandages on

---

[13] Drobot and Thom

[14] Vieira, C. et al.

for 24 hours unless you have an adverse reaction, such as itching or burning, in which case remove the bandage and wash the area with soap and water. When you remove the bandage after 24 hours, if there is no visible rash or irritation it is safe for you to use castor oil topically.

Because some people experience a mild sedative effect from castor oil packs, we recommend doing them just before sleep when possible.

These suggestions, taught and used in sexological bodywork, were originally developed by Edgar Cayce.

You will need:

1. Organic, cold-pressed castor oil

2. A hot water bottle (or two)

3. Plastic wrap

4. Three one-foot square pieces of organic wool or organic cotton flannel, or one piece large enough to cover the entire abdomen when folded in thirds

5. One large old bath towel

How to Make and Use a Castor Oil Pack

- Fold the flannel in thirds so it is still large enough to fit over your entire abdomen but is now three layers thick, or stack the three squares.

- Drizzle the room temperature oil over one side of the flannel as if you are icing a cake. Drizzle in multiple directions and really soak the flannel with the oil.

- Lie on your back and place the oiled side of the flannel

directly onto your abdomen; cover the flannel with the sheet of plastic (you may chose to do these two steps while standing and wrap the plastic wrap around your body to "hold" the flannel in place), and place the hot water bottle on top of the plastic wrap.

- Cover everything with the old towel to insulate the heat. (Please note that castor oil can stain. Take caution not to get the oil on whatever you are laying on, and, if necessary, cover that surface with something to protect it.)

- Leave pack on for 60 minutes. Some people recommend elevating your feet during this time (using a pillow under your knees and feet works well). Feel free to do so if it feels more comfortable or pleasurable.

- When finished, remove the layers of the pack. Fold the flannel with the castor oil side facing in and store the pack in a large zip-lock bag or other plastic container until your next use. You can reuse the flannel up to seven times; simply add more oil (drizzling like you are decorating a cake) each time. The pack will become more saturated with each use. Dispose of the flannel after one full week of use (it can not be washed and re-used), or sooner if desired.

- You can wash the oil from your skin using a solution of two tablespoons of baking soda to one quart water, or just soap and water. If you do the castor oil pack before bed, you may want to just leave the oil on your skin overnight. The oil will likely stain the clothes you sleep in that night, so be sure to choose something you are willing to have stained.

- Be careful when laundering the towel wrapped on top of the pack or the nightclothes you sleep in after the pack. It is recommended that you wash these items separately from other laundry as the castor oil can make other clothes smell like castor oil if washed together.

There are a variety of recommendations for duration and frequency of castor oil pack use. Ask your body which schedule feels right to you. Or, honestly and without self-judgment, assess which schedule feels the most easeful and pleasurable for you to commit to so that you can successfully complete the course of treatment.

- One week: Apply daily

- One month: Apply four consecutive days in each week

- One month: Apply three times a week for three of the weeks in the month, taking one week off at some point in the month.

Exercises

We offer some general exercises that help with building awareness of the pelvic floor while relieving chronic tension. Exercises to address persistent pelvic pain usually do not involve strengthening, toning and tightening. We want to create a felt sense and a visualization of the pelvis that can assist us in moving with somatic awareness, while inviting increased flexibility, stability, mobility and choice. People should see a physiotherapist for help with getting exercises to target the specific areas and muscles involved in their particular form of pelvic pain.

Fascial Stretch

You can feel and heal your own fascial network through stretching. Try tuning in and allowing your body to find its preferred stretches. Slowly unwind your body from the pelvic bowl. Expand your length and breadth, feeling your bones lengthen and your muscles slide across one another. When you come to a stopping point in your stretch, stretch into it for awhile. After 60-90 seconds of holding the stretch at the "resilient edge of resistance," you might feel a fascial release, and continue unwinding.

Pelvic Bowl Dancing

The pelvis moves in many directions.

Figure 25: In the saggital plane the pelvis moves forward and backwards

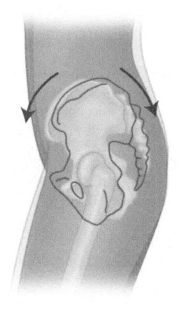

Figure 26: In the frontal plane the pelvis moves up and down

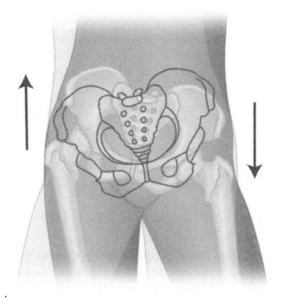

Figure 27: In the horizontal plane, the pelvis rotates in and out.

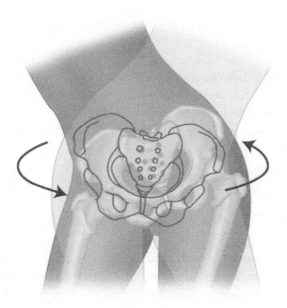

All these movements can be combined as you imagine carrying water and sloshing water in your pelvic bowl. Put on some music and dance and enjoy tracking how the water is sloshing in your pelvic bowl as you move your hips. Move your bowl in, out, up, down, and round and round. Move side to side, tilt, rotate, and see how many ways you can move the bowl.

"Kiss the Earth" Breath

Sitting down on a chair or a cushion, bring your attention to the weight of your pelvis, held by gravity. Breath slowly and deeply, with awareness of the pelvic diaphragm. Focus now on your anus. Feel or imagine your anus open, soften and kiss the earth with every inbreath. Feel any sensation in the nerves of the anal area, charged and enlivened with your breath and awareness.

Pucker up by giving your anal sphincter muscles a little squeeze with your outbreath. Feel or imagine sensation, pumping energy from the anus through the whole body. Feel or imagine the electrical currents traveling through the nerves. Notice and name any sensations.

Stay with this awareness of your anus as it kisses the earth. Breathe in with a kiss, breathe out to send energy from the kiss through your whole body. Allow yourself to get curious. Can you enjoy the sensations? Can you feel yourself connected more deeply to the earth with every breath?

Pelvic Tilts

Lie on your back with your knees bent, feet on the floor. Spend some time here with your spine in neutral, and the sacrum, not the lower back, resting on the floor. Breathe deeply. Hold your pelvis stable while you breathe.

Then on the outbreath, cinch your waist at the end of the exhalation. Press your spine into the floor. Notice the pelvis tilt backwards. Hold for five seconds. On the in breath, allow the spine to curve away from the floor, the front hip bones release upwards, the tailbone moves into the floor. Hold for five seconds. Return to neutral spine. Stay there for awhile, noticing.

Figure 28:Pelvic tilts

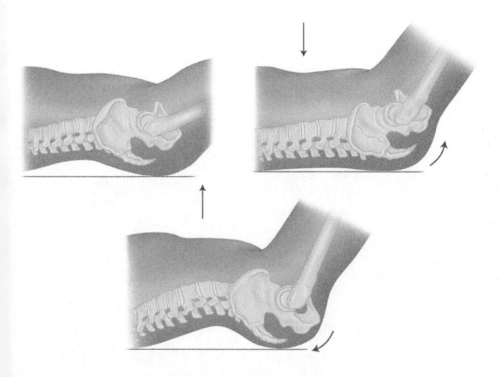

Squats

Squats stretch the pelvic floor. Relaxing while lingering in a nice wide squat can help our muscles change and ease their tension patterns.

A "squatty potty" is helpful. The muscles of the pelvic floor that constrict to hold in our poo can ease when we are in a squat. They cannot release fully when we simply sit.

You can gently build capacity for squatting by doing wall squats. Lean against a wall, heels about 18 inches from it. Slowly slide down into the depth of squat that gently stretches your personal comfort zone. Hold for 5-10 seconds and come back up.

Figure 29: Wide-legged squats stretch the pelvic floor

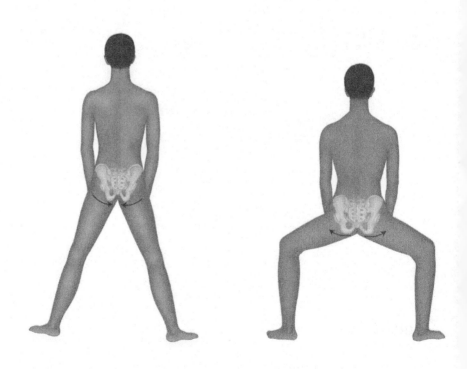

Hump and Hollow

On your hands and knees, relax your abdomen and let your back sag downward and your tail stick up. Then hump your back, tucking in your tail. Find the in-between space of neutral spine, where your tail is neither tucked in nor sticking up. Breathe into this place of ease, noticing.

Figure 30: Hump and hollow

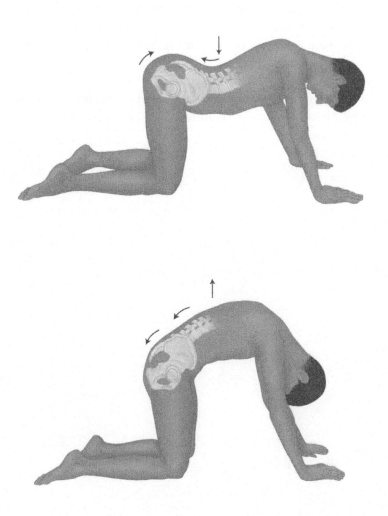

Elevator

Think of your external sphincter muscles as the main floor. Gently squeeze the muscles you use to stop from pooing and peeing. Then squeeze and lift the elevator all the way up to the pelvic diaphragm. Stop as if your elevator has made it up to the second floor. Now a little bit higher. Bring your gentle squeeze the muscles in the upper part of your pelvic bowl. Now the most important part - Relax. Feel the relaxation as the elevator goes back down very, very slowly. Stop at the second floor. Relax the muscles all the way. Then slowly, slowly down again. Relax the tension in your sphincter muscles. Then imagine letting go even more, slowly going all the way down into the basement. Imagine the doors slide open - releasing every last bit of tension with this image. Really breathe into the ease of complete relaxation, or as complete as it can be, in this moment. Now start the elevator again and bring it up, slowly, stopping and noticing at each floor.

Figure 31: Schematic frontal cross section showing levels of muscles in the pelvic diaphragm

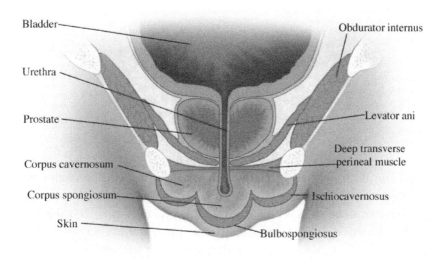

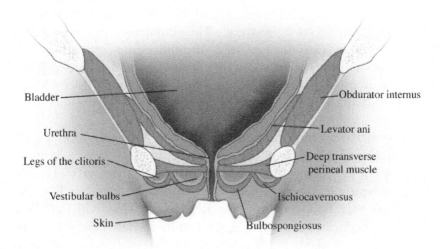

Beyond Pain to Pleasure

The medical model of addressing pelvic pain often fails to realize that the absence of pain is not the same as the presence of pleasure. We've known clients who have worked for years to resolve their pain conditions through physical therapy or other traditional bodywork modalities, only to discover once they were free of pain that they still were not experiencing pleasure. So after all those years of hard work, it was "back to the drawing board" with this new "problem". As somatic sex educators supporting somatic awareness, we simultaneously cultivate a relationship with our pain *and* our pleasure (and all the sensations in between). The abundance of nerves in our pelvis means it can be a source of both. Engaging in somatic awareness will bring us into more awareness of and dialogue with our pain, but it will also create the opportunity for us to discover and interact with our pleasure.

It is incredibly important for people living with pain to find ways to connect with pleasure in their bodies. Pain can completely hijack our awareness, leading us to believe that is all there is to be felt. Shauna identifies as experiencing mild chronic pain in her life, and she discovered that was true for her. In working with a fellow somatic sex educator at a training, she commented that the rocks hurt her feet as she walked, and her colleague reflected, "So you orient to the pain in your body first". She was stunned, never having realized that when checking in with her body, the first—and often only—sensations she noticed were painful ones. This tendency or habit is exacerbated when our pain is not mild. But with gentle practice we can discover and cultivate the many sensations in our body, not just our pain.

Try this: Allow yourself to settle into a comfortable position, whatever that is for you. Ask yourself, "What is the most pleasurable place in my body right now?" and drop inside to notice. Maybe you notice that spot right away. If not, allow your attention to rove your body, seeking even the tiniest place of pleasure. Once you find it, let your attention gently rest there for at least 10-20 seconds if you can. Your pain might snag your attention, which is fine. Acknowledge the pain sensation and then direct your attention back to that pleasurable spot. If you absolutely can not find a place of pleasure—which happens!—scan your body slowly and discern the least uncomfortable place. Rest your attention there briefly, noticing the sensations, and then give yourself a break. Play with this game as often as you like.

This exploration may bring to awareness the habit of choosing touch that addresses pain, such as asking your partner to massage or stroke a painful place. This is great, of course, and can bring some relief to our painful places. But consider occasionally asking (of your partner or yourself) for touch that is solely about pleasure, not about the pleasure of somewhat easing your pain. Again feel into that pleasurable (or least uncomfortable place) in your body. Now reflect what kind of touch there would feel great. Ask for that touch or give it to yourself.

Engaging in "pleasure practices" is not about denying or ignoring your pain. Quite the opposite. It's a both/and practice, not an either/or practice. Cultivating pleasure while we work to address pain is about harnessing the incredible power of pleasure as a resource for our healing journey. It actively supports our brain in cultivating neural pathways that allow us to feel pleasure, while it weakens the pathways dedicated to our pain.

When we focus our attention on pleasure, we are literally rewiring our nervous system, including our brain, to increase our capacity for pleasure. The fancy word for this is neuroplasticity, but it's easily understood with a "garden path" analogy. If you walk through a garden, following the same path every day, you'll wear that path into the earth more and more deeply over time. It gets easier and easier to stay on that path—or rather, you get less and less likely to wander off of it. Like that garden path, our nervous system functions using neural pathways. Neurons that get used repeatedly stay connected in networks, aka neural pathways. Neural pathways that don't get used, get pruned. Imagine that one day in your garden, you take a different route. Maybe it's the most pleasurable walk you've ever had in your garden. If you never walk that way again, there won't be any record of your most pleasurable walk. The grass grows strong again, the flowers that bent as you passed them straighten up. Nature fills in the temporary "groove" you made in the garden and that pathway is no longer visible. Our nervous system prunes rarely used pathways just like nature fills them in in the garden.

When we mindfully focus on pleasure, we are strengthening "pleasure grooves" in our nervous system. We are literally increasing our capacity for pleasure by creating new pleasure pathways in our body. We are also working to compensate for our brain's negativity bias. Our brain really does naturally focus on pain, which it perceives as a message of danger. We've all noticed this bias throughout our lives. "Why can't I remember the good things as well as I remember the bad things?" A negativity bias makes sense inasmuch as paying attention to what is dangerous protects us from further harm. But this bias is bad news for those of us living with chronic pain. We can work to contradict the brain's built-in negativity bias by deepening our pleasure grooves, increasing our neural capacity for pleasure. Researchers have documented that positive or pleasurable experiences must be focused on for 10-20 seconds to become a memory. So slow down, savor those pleasurable moments, and know that you are slowly but surely rewiring your nervous system by doing so.[15]

Unfortunately, building these pleasure pathways doesn't happen with one experience of 10-20 seconds of focused attention; rewiring the nervous system requires consistent practice over time. Think of that garden path: the more often you walk it, weed it, care for it and

---

[15] This paragraph draws on the work of Rick Hanson

pay attention, the more established it becomes. No one learns to play an instrument or speak a language in one practice session. All embodied or somatic learning and transformation requires conscious practice over time. We're slowly feeling our way into a new way of being—one of less pain and more pleasure. Stepping into a new way of being is no small project! Be patient with yourself and just keep practicing.

Physical pain also impacts us emotionally and spiritually, and those impacts don't just disappear even if physical symptoms can be completely resolved. Even if we cultivate our physical awareness of and capacity for pleasure with diligence, we may need additional work and play to reconnect with the emotional and spiritual aspects of pleasure and eroticism. This has certainly been true for Caffyn, whose long journey with pelvic pain both stemmed from and led to painful relational experiences. They are continually unfolding the pleasures of more trust, communication, connection and reverence in body, spirit and relationships.

Shauna discovered the disconnect between physical healing and emotional and spiritual healing during her recovery from nervous system collapse. Both depression and the drugs used to treat it had tremendous negative impacts on her sexuality and sexual expression. When she finally found a treatment that didn't involve sexual side-effects and recovered to a place where her body once again functioned sexually, she noticed that she was still avoiding sex and intimacy, even with herself. She wrote on her blog:

> I've been waiting to just suddenly feel like "my old (sexual) self" again. But I'm not my old self. I'm the me who has been through a year and a half of illness and recovery, with all the incredible learning and the unfortunate baggage that comes with that. I'm going to have to accept that I've been impacted emotionally, spiritually, psychologically, that just fixing the physiology of eroticism doesn't automatically make all that go away. I'm going to have to *choose* to engage with my sexuality to bring it fully back online. I'm going to have to court her, like two lovers coming back together after each have been off on separate adventures. People who have been

changed by their experiences but are still committed to being in relationship, and who choose to feel into a new dynamic of connection. Maybe even one that is more fulfilling, more satisfying than before.

People often report feeling abandoned after completing treatment in the standard medical model, released into the world with a "You're cured! Good luck!" and left to figure out how to integrate their experience and move forward in their lives on their own. We recognize that your physiological healing is only one aspect of recovery, and we encourage you to get support for all aspects of your experience and healing – body, mind and soul.

Staying Connected to Sexual Pleasure with Persistent Pelvic Pain

Redefining Sex

How can people dealing with persistent pelvic pain stay connected to their eroticism and continue to enjoy and nourish erotic partnerships? The first step is redefining sex. When we understand "sex" as "penetrative intercourse culminating in orgasm" we have a very impoverished definition of sex. This definition robs everyone of pleasure and the joy of full sexual expression. We are not recommending redefining sex because pelvic pain prevents us from having "real" sex. Quite the opposite! Supporting people to expand their definition of what constitutes sex is foundational to our work as sex educators. We suggest that everyone, regardless of pain or health status, let go of any ideas of what sex is "supposed" to look like and follow their pleasure instead. Below are a number of strategies to explore, both with yourself and/or your partner(s), as you expand your sexual repertoire and discover ways to access pleasure without triggering pain.

Explore pleasure with relaxation or lower levels of arousal

Sexual experiences do not have to follow an arc of constantly building arousal (and tension) leading to climax. In fact, bringing more relaxation and savoring of sensation into our arousal patterns is a technique for increasing the amount of pleasure we are capable of experiencing. By slowing down, you can actually increase your capacity to feel pleasure! Arousal is a dance between tension and relaxation, excitement and savoring. Engage the dance. It's common for people to tense the muscles of their bodies as their arousal builds. Begin to notice when you start to tense any muscles in your body. Pause and consciously relax your entire body. Then resume the stimulation, allowing arousal to build while trying to keep the body relaxed. When you notice tension returning to the muscles, pause again. Relax your body, savor what you are noticing and then repeat.

Notice and engage your breath as you explore relaxed arousal. Occasionally take a slow, deep breath; imagine the sexual energy or pleasure you are building expands throughout your body as you inhale and allow your body to relax as you exhale.

Explore the sensual

Get creative with different kinds of touch or different objects that can create a variety of sensations for your body. Feathers, fur, and fabrics of different textures are classic choices. Brushes offer an endless variety of sensations: paintbrushes, a silicone basting brush, an electric toothbrush or any number of textures of hairbrushes. Play with temperature, ice cubes and candle wax being classic choices. Consider a cool metal spoon, a stone warmed in hot water, or a spritz of water from a spray bottle out of the fridge. Get creative! What about a sharp-toothed comb or the fringe on a jacket? Take a stroll through a dollar store or hardware store with an eye for things that might feel good on your body.

Kink and Power Play

BDSM, kink, role play, power play. There are a lot of words applied to this very broad and diverse realm of erotic practices, many of which don't require any kind of touch while still offering access to erotic pleasure and partner connection. See the bibliography for recommendations on beginner-friendly books on the subject(s).

Pelvic Pain and Partnership

Pelvic pain often impacts our partners and relationships, and the stress of that can certainly add to the overall stress of the situation, which exacerbates physical pain. It's important to acknowledge this stress, and to stay in communication with your partner(s) about what's going on for you. The vulnerability of sex can cause people to take things personally, even when it really has nothing to do with them, and partners can sometimes feel rejected in the face of your pain if they're not kept in the loop. Acknowledging that your pain impacts your partner does not in any way make it "your fault". Work together to find ways to stay intimately connected that feel good to both of you. When genital touch isn't an option, what kind of touch *would* feel good? Would it feel good to cuddle, clothed or naked? Would it feel good to have them stroke your head or give you a massage? What if you tried to recreate those early years of dating, when you would make out for hours and just savor the pleasure in your body without it going "beyond" making out? What if you held your partner in some way while they masturbated, maybe whispering sexy things in their ear the whole time? Consider visiting a sex store (or "visit" one online) or go see a sex coach to get new ideas for ways to play sexually with your partner(s). Check out "adult games" or books that provide ideas for partnered erotic explorations that can really help expand your vocabulary of erotic play.

Mindful Masturbation

Mindfully engaging in regular self-pleasuring practice can contribute to the management or banishment of pelvic pain.

People often masturbate in habitual, efficient ways. And in the presence of persistent pelvic pain, people sometimes extinguish sexual feeling, and may even forgo masturbating altogether. We suggest bringing a dedicated self-pleasure practice into our lives. With creative touch techniques, extended time devoted to masturbation, and mindful attention to body sensation, we can learn to enjoy erotic aliveness in various stages of arousal. We can notice more easily when pleasure turns to pain, or when pain coexists with pleasure. And the more we foster pleasure, even in small ways, the more we can welcome pleasure into our pelvis.

As we explored in the chapter "Beyond Pain to Pleasure," we literally change our nervous system through the practice of pleasure. Neuropsychologist Rick Hanson suggests three steps for cultivating happiness that can be fruitfully applied to mindful masturbation. We cultivate neuroplastic change in this way:

1. Observe.

2. Pull weeds.

3. Plant flowers

On the first point, we can **observe** and learn to be with all that is, within and without. Observe yourself and your unique erotic ecosystem with compassionate kindness. Your personal history, inborn tendencies, and the different natural and human communities you live in all shape the garden of your erotic wellbeing. Notice what brings you pleasure in small and large ways: physical, emotional, mental and spiritual. Notice what you are grateful for. Notice body sensation.

On the second point, we **pull weeds** by reducing shame, self-judgment, and negative thoughts. Notice negative or catastrophic thinking about yourself and your body, relationships (or the absence of relationships), access (or lack of access) to orgasm, use (or lack of use) of toys, porn, fantasy. 'Pulling weeds' doesn't mean you need to lose weight, get a better relationship, have more orgasms, and stop using porn. Our *negative thoughts* are the weeds in our erotic garden. It is our *shame* about erotic life that diminishes us, rather than any aspect of erotic life itself. Pull weeds by gently observing your negative self-judgments and releasing them with loving kindness, refocusing on what is positive and pleasurable now.

On the third point, we can **plant** what we want to harvest. Each person's garden can produce beautiful nourishing foods of pleasure. So plant more joy by dreaming into what you want for yourself and your erotic life. Plant the seeds, and provide, as best you can, the conditions for your vision to flourish. Savoring the process will best prepare you for harvesting the ripe fruit. Choose pleasure in small and large ways. Practice and savour pleasure.

Make Room for Resistance

Sometimes we find we can't sustain focus, can't enjoy self-pleasure sessions, hurt too much, can't connect with our erotic energy, or simply can't make time. If you are in a place or time when mindful masturbation is hard for you, don't get hard on yourself about it. See if you can come from a place of self-kindness to find what works, start again tomorrow, or just give yourself some space to do what really brings you authentic pleasure today.

Bibliography and Resources

Almaas, A.H. *The Void: Inner Spaciousness and Ego Structure.* Shambala, 2000.

Barral, J.-P., 1993. *Urogenital Manipulation*, English ed. edition. ed. Eastland Press Inc, Seattle.

Barral. J.P. *Manual Therapy for the Prostate,* North Atlantic Books, 2010

Barnes, John. The Fascial Pelvis. Massage Magazine October 2008, p. 68-71

Berceli, D., 2008. *The Revolutionary Trauma Release Process: Transcend Your Toughest Times.* Namaste Publishing, Vancouver.

Blum, Charles L. The relationship between the pelvis and stomatognathic system: a position statement. Journal of Vertebral Subluxation Research, March 3, 2010, pages 1-3

Calais-Germain, B., 2003. *The Female Pelvis Anatomy & Exercises,* Ill edition. ed. Eastland Press, Seattle, WA.

Carter, M. & L., 2015. *Completely Overcome Vaginismus: The Practical Approach to Pain-Free Intercourse.* www.vaginismus.com

Cutler, N., Bodyworker's Pearl: The Jaw and Hip Connection | Massage Professionals Update [WWW Document]. URL https://www.integrativehealthcare.org/mt/archives/2010/06/bodyworkers_pea.html (accessed 5.14.18).

England, P. and R. Horowitz. *Birthing From Within.* Partera Press, Albuquerque, 1998

Fischer, M.J., Riedlinger, K., Gutenbrunner, C., Bernateck, M., 2009. Influence of the temporomandibular joint on range of motion of the hip joint in patients with complex regional pain syndrome. J Manipulative Physiol Ther 32, 364–371. https://doi.org/10.1016/j.jmpt.2009.04.003

Forsberg, M., n.d. The Mysterious Relationship of Pelvis and Jaw [WWW Document]. Align PT Longmont Boulder Manual Physical Therapy. URL https://www.alignpt.com/single-post/2017/01/05/The-Mysterious-Relationship-of-Pelvis-and-Jaw (accessed 5.14.18).

Franklin, E., 2003. *Pelvic Power: Mind/Body Exercises for Strength, Flexibility, Posture, and Balance for Men and Women*, 1 edition. ed. Elysian Editions, Highstown, NJ.

Hanson, R., 2013. *Hardwiring Happiness: The New Brain Science of Contentment, Calm, and Confidence*. Harmony, New York.

Howard, Leslie, 2017. *Pelvic Liberation: Using Yoga, Self-Inquiry, and Breath Awareness for Pelvic Health*. Leslie Howard Yoga.

Jeoff Drobot,, Thom Dickson, n.d. Castor Oil: An Essential for Health | Marion Institute [WWW Document]. URL https://www.marioninstitute.org/castor-oil-an-essential-for-health/ (accessed 5.14.18).

Jesse, C., 2016. *Science for Sexual Happiness: A Guide to Reclaiming Erotic Pleasure*. erospirit.

Jesse, C., 2015. *Erotic Massage for Healing and Pleasure: plus Orgasm Coaching, Genital Anatomy, Scar Tissue Healing and more from a pioneering Somatic Sex Educator*. erospirit.

Kent, Tami Lynne, 2011. *Wild Feminine: Finding Power, Spirit & Joy in the Female Body*. Atria Books/Beyond Words

Krause, M., Wheeler, T.L., Richter, H.E., Snyder, T.E., 2010. Systemic Effects of Vaginally Administered Estrogen Therapy: A Review. Female Pelvic Med Reconstr Surg 16, 188–195. https://doi.org/10.1097/SPV.0b013e3181d7e86e

Levine, P.A., 2008. *Healing Trauma: A Pioneering Program for Restoring the Wisdom of Your Body*, Pap/Com edition. ed. Sounds True, Boulder, Colo.; Enfield.

Lowen, A., 1994. *Bioenergetics: The Revolutionary Therapy That Uses the Language of the Body to Heal the Problems of the Mind*, New edition edition. ed. Penguin, New York.

Meltzer-Brody, S., Leserman, J., Zolnoun, D., Steege, J., Green, E., Teich, A., 2007. Trauma and posttraumatic stress disorder in women with chronic pelvic pain. Obstet Gynecol 109, 902–908. https://doi.org/10.1097/01.AOG.0000258296.35538.88

Morpheus. *How to be Kinky: A Beginners Guide to BDSM*.

National Institute of Diabetes and Digestive and Kidney Diseases, n.d. Abdominal Adhesions | NIDDK [WWW Document]. URL https://www.niddk.nih.gov/health-information/digestive-diseases/abdominal-adhesions (accessed 4.27.18).

Network, W.H., n.d. Treatments For Vaginal Dryness – Women's Health Network [WWW Document]. URL https://www.womenshealthnetwork.com/sexandfertility/treatmentsforvaginaldryness.aspx (accessed 4.27.18).

Taormino, Tristan. *The Ultimate Guide to Kink: BDSM, Role Play and the Erotic Edge.*

Therapies: Castor Oil Packs [WWW Document], n.d. URL https://www.edgarcayce.org/the-readings/health-and-wellness/holistic-health-database/therapies-castor-oil-packs/ (accessed 5.14.18).

van der Kolk, B., 2002. Posttraumatic Therapy in the Age of Neuroscience: *Psychoanalytic Dialogues:* Vol 12, No 3 [WWW Document]. URL https://www.tandfonline.com/doi/abs/10.1080/10481881209348674 (accessed 5.14.18).

van der Kolk, B., 2015. *The Body Keeps the Score: Brain, Mind, and Body in the Healing of Trauma.* Penguin Books.

Vieira, C., Evangelista, S., Cirillo, R., Lippi, A., Maggi, C.A., Manzini, S., 2000. Effect of ricinoleic acid in acute and subchronic experimental models of inflammation. Mediators Inflamm 9, 223–228.

Wise, D., Ph D., Anderson, R.U., Ph D. *A Headache in the Pelvis: A New Understanding and Treatment for Prostatitis and Chronic Pelvic Pain Syndromes.* Natl Center for Pelvic Pain, Occidental, 2003

About the Authors

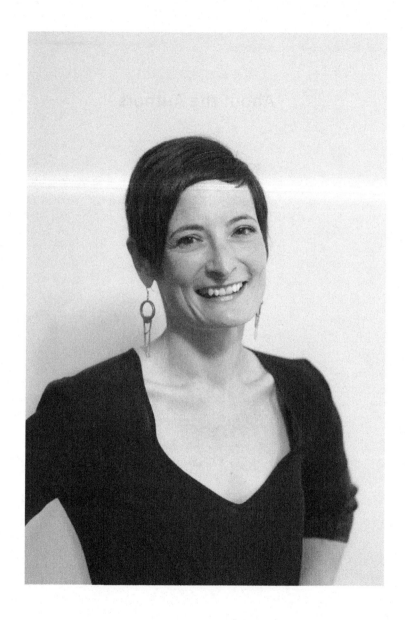

Shauna Farabaugh is a certified Somatic Sex Educator and certified Tension and Trauma Releasing Exercises (TRE®) provider who fiercely believes in the right to sexual expression for *every body* and is committed to making sex education "sexcessible" for all. She is particularly passionate about supporting clients who find themselves at the intersection between their sexuality and life transitions of all kinds—both how life change impacts sexual identity and expression and how to connect with our sexuality in times of transition as a source of strength, resilience and wisdom to guide us through change. Illness, injury, surgery, pelvic pain, grief, loss, cancer treatment, childbirth – Shauna supports clients to integrate, evolve, and thrive, harnessing the power of transition to allow for transformation, and to come out more embodied and sexier than ever on the other side of life's transitions.

Shauna has been a professional sex educator for over a decade, working in school districts, disability service organizations, and private practice. She has earned certifications from San Francisco Sex Information, The Institute for the Advanced Study of Human Sexuality, and the Somatic Sex Educators Association. She serves as adjunct faculty at the Institute for the Study of Somatic Sexology. She is also a founding member of the Bay Area Sexuality and Disability Network.

Reverently irreverent, Shauna brings a profound sense of play to both her group classes and one on one work with clients of all genders, sexualities, and sexual lifestyles…because sex really is supposed to be fun!

See her website at www.sexualityintransition.com

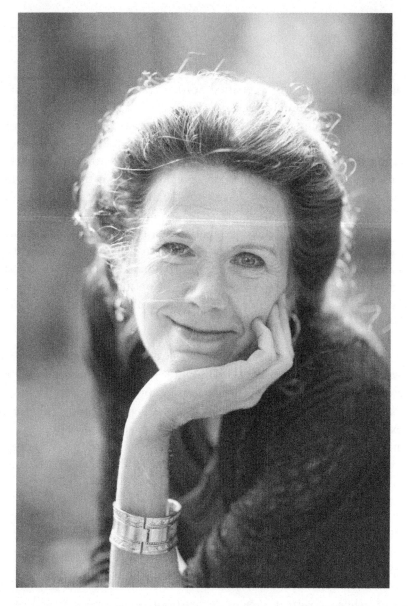

Encouraging neuroplastic change to support sexual healing and expanded pleasure, unwinding sexual trauma, honoring the gender galaxy, exploring the intersection of sex and spirit, creating erotic community – **Caffyn Jesse** welcomes people from around the world to personal sessions and workshops at their Salt Spring Island studio. They offer free and paid teachings online.

Caffyn teaches the Sexological Bodywork and Somatic Sex Education professional trainings in Canada. They offer a weeklong training for Intimacy Educators at their Salt Spring Island studio, plus occasional workshops on somatic sex education topics ranging from pelvic pain to sex in long-term relationships. They have a trauma training for professionals who touch.

People of all gender identities and sexual orientations are welcomed and celebrated in Caffyn's sessions, classes and workshops.

Caffyn has researched and written on the science of somatic sex education, neurobiology and sexual healing, trauma, orgasm coaching and many other topics. Their books include *Science for Sexual Happiness* and *Erotic Massage for Healing and Pleasure*. Video programs include *Healing Circumcision: Work with Scars* (which is available free on their website), *Learn Erotic Massage* and *Breathe the Body Erotic*.

See their website at www.erospirit.ca

Made in the USA
Monee, IL
06 January 2021

56495864R00062